Sweaty, Sore, Sometimes *Hungry*

Sweaty, Sore, Sometimes *Hungry*

The Painful Joys of a Living Sacrifice

MARVIN GILBERT

RESOURCE *Publications* · Eugene, Oregon

Resource Publications
An Imprint of Wipf and Stock Publishers
199 W. 8th Ave., Suite 3
Eugene, OR 97401

www.wipfandstock.com

PAPERBACK ISBN: 978-1-5326-6606-3
HARDCOVER ISBN: 978-1-5326-6607-0
EBOOK ISBN: 978-1-5326-6608-7

Manufactured in the U.S.A.   01/10/19

Contents

Appendices

List of Tables

Preface

IN LATE 2011, I embarked on a unique (for me) health journey that continues to deeply impact my life. I abandoned the traditional three meals a day and began eating only when I was actually hungry. Distinguishing between true hunger and clock-dictated habit took some time. Largely by accident, I discovered that my morning coffee, followed by an hour of fairly intense exercise in the gym, pushed back true hunger for hours. Eventually this and related discoveries shaped my current two-meals-a-day pattern of eating: a late morning brunch and a modest evening meal. I adopted this pattern long before I learned that this is termed "intermittent fasting" in the fitness literature.

Sweaty, Sore, Sometimes Hungry, in part, describes the physical and spiritual transformation I began at age 63. This is not an autobiography, however. The book's diverse chapters argue consistently for the pursuit of holistic health. Essentially, these sixteen chapters challenge readers to get off of the couch, purchase the gym membership and training shoes, and love God authentically—as whole, faithful stewards of the bodies he entrusted to their care.

This book also builds the case that suffering is normative for Christians. Suffering is neither evidence of God's displeasure nor of their own failure. Similarly, pain is not a horror to be avoided at all costs; it can, in fact, coexist with deep and abiding joy. By welcoming suffering, we can reunite body and spirit in the gym and in the fast. The discipline demanded in the gym is essentially the same required during an extended fast. Great rewards await those willing to endure discipline's pain for the sake of entering their Master's joy (Matt 25:23).

I owe a deep debt of gratitude to my wife, Rosie; this is a better book because of her careful proofreading. I also appreciate the feedback my children gave to an earlier version of the manuscript; their influence is reflected throughout. And I am so grateful for the creativity of Kelvin Co; his original images appearing in the five unit introductions are amazing. My deepest debt of gratitude, however, is reserved for my Lord. How patiently he has led me into integrated, holistic health! Like the psalmist, I bear witness to the amazing impact of his steadfast love: it does, indeed, endure forever (Ps 100:5).

Introduction

SWEATY, SORE, SOMETIMES HUNGRY is intended to function as a wake-up call for those Christians who rarely, if ever, train their bodies or restrain their appetites. It will also serve as a resource—hopefully an inspirational one—for those who already know the "painful joys" of self-discipline in both the gym and the "closet" of private fasting.

The first two chapters, composing Unit 1, examine the biblical foundation for viewing our bodies as treasures entrusted to our care. For reasons that still amaze me, God longs to dwell *with* us and *in* us—in our bodies! Anything that diminishes his welcome in us is sinful. In this context, Chapter 1 argues that the "Great Divide" between body and spirit (the Divide most Christians accept as normative) is heresy. God designed us to be whole beings, living to *"the praise of his glory"* (Eph 1:12) with both our spirits *and* our bodies. Thus, we must steward our bodies well, valuing them as treasures entrusted to our care. Elaborating on this theme, chapter 2 reminds readers that God will hold us accountable for the quality of our stewardship.

Unit 2, *Sweaty*, explores in four chapters the nature of, and strategies for achieving, cardiovascular fitness. These chapters consistently argue that moderation is the key to sustainable cardio exercise. Too much, too fast *always* kills motivation. Sustained efforts in elevating our heart rates for *at least* two hours a week bear lasting fruit. Minutes do matter: chapter 3 demonstrates how the minutes we invest in physical fitness add up to cardiovascular health over time.

The three chapters in Unit 3, *Sore*, focus on the contribution of strength training to the enhancement of personal discipline and holistic wellbeing. As is true of cardo training, strength training thrives on consistent goal-focused commitment. Chapter 8 explains that when we demand more effort from our muscles than they are accustomed to delivering, they become sore. Those sore muscles are evidence that we are growing stronger: able to lift at some future point more than we ever thought was possible prior to the effort . . . and prior to the goal-setting that motivated that effort. Constantly asking questions about our performance, introduced in chapter 9, enhances motivation and creates new possibilities of strength-training success.

Chapters 10 through 13 (Unit 4, *Sometimes Hungry*) shift the readers' focus from the busy gym to the empty plate. Jesus prophesied-promised that his disciples *would* fast after he returned to the Father (Matt 9:15). Fasting uniquely merges physical and spiritual disciplines. In moderation, fasting works wonders; only fasting can break the idolatrous power of food *and* renew us at the cellular level. Fasting also allows us—at a very mild level—to enter into our Lord's suffering. Many believers eagerly long to know Christ in the awesome *"power of his resurrection."* Far fewer, it seems, long to *"share his sufferings"* (Phil 3:10). Fasting transforms this latter goal into a gut-level reality.

Unit 5, *Painful Joys,* argues across its three chapters that pain is unavoidable, beginning the day of our birth. Chapter 14 notes that pain-free living is a delusional and ultimately self-destructive goal. And as explained in chapter 15, what has amazed me, in the context of my cancer treatment that began in 2014, is that pain and joy can paradoxically coexist within the believer. Even as pain pulls us close to the Father's open heart, joy erupts within our souls during that journey.

Sweaty, Sore, Sometimes Hungry concludes with an emphasis on a radical New Testament concept: God now demands *human,* not animal, sacrifices! As God's *living* sacrifices, we are challenged daily to *"glorify God"* in our bodies (1 Cor 6:20), and to do so *"with joy that is inexpressible and filled with glory"* (1 Pet 1:8).

UNIT 1
Biblical Foundations

Chapter 1: Healing the Heretical Divide: Reuniting Body and Spirit
Chapter 2: Living as a Grateful Steward: Harmonizing Gift and Responsibility

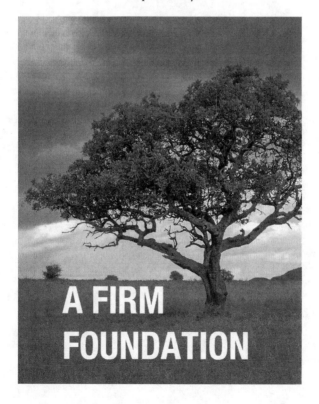

1

Healing the Heretical Divide
Reuniting Body and Spirit

"The glory of God is man fully alive." Irenaeus of Lyon[1]

DESTRUCTIVE DIVISION

WE ARE DIVIDED! NOT just a little bit; we are *deeply* divided, and have been so since birth. This internal Great Divide is as real as Adam and Eve's ejection from the Garden of Eden. The perfect physical and spiritual unity known only by our first parents was brutally ruptured at the Fall. And it remains ruptured—badly so—in all of us! Such is the destructive nature of sin.

This division of body and spirit[2] is so severe most of us never fully recover from it—at least not during this life. The Great Divide reveals itself in diverse, but always destructive ways. For example, some people who once publicly pledged to live together faithfully now privately consume pornography whenever possible. And

1. http://www.ewtn.com/library/theology/irenaeus.htm.

2. I use the term *spirit* in a general sense: that which is immaterial (non-corporeal) in us; this includes the soul.

3

morbidly obese Christians, committed to living under Christ's Lordship and discipline, waddle home each week from their favorite all-you-can-eat Sunday buffets.

The Great Divide marks us all in profound ways. Most spiritual shepherds—some ironically modelling the problem in their own lifestyles and waistlines—simply avoid this risk-filled topic. This irony becomes intensely uncomfortable if they ever preach from 1 Corinthians 6:19–20[3] (and similar verses). Their intense discomfort with such passages, perhaps, explains why those texts are so rarely preached.

SECULAR OBSESSION WITH SPIRITUALITY AND WHOLENESS

A few decades ago, Eastern religions and cults began gaining popularity in the West. Western societies in general began a related shift from a God-is-essential spirituality to a humanism-is-enough secular spirituality. Now, odd-looking gurus publically laud their money-making goal of "wholeness" without offering a credible solution to the Great Divide. Oprah and others have popularized this logically absurd concept while emphasizing the amazing power of human effort.

Without question, this secular pursuit of "spirituality" is broadly appealing. In essence, it promises, yet is unable to deliver, personal wholeness and health. The spiritual rupture that violently tore through the Garden continues to dominate our fragmented lives, despite our best efforts to "reintegrate" ourselves. Talk show hosts, pop psychologists, and Eastern gurus can *never* offer the path to true inner wholeness.[4] The Great Divide is too deep, too pervasive to be mended through human effort.

---

3. This passage is quoted at the end of this chapter. All Scripture quotations, unless otherwise stated, are from the English Standard Version.

4. The power of sin, reflecting the full impact of the fall, condemns to failure all such humanistic efforts.

HERETICAL EMBRACE OF THE GREAT DIVIDE

Reality whispers persistently that all human efforts to heal the Great Divide of body and spirit fail miserably. Pastors highlight this fact, while ironically proclaiming a diminished or truncated version of the gospel that focuses only on the sinner's *spiritual* divide from the Creator. And, admirably, many Christians seek to win "souls," knowing that *"he who wins souls is wise"* (Prov 11:30, NKJV). Yet most pastors remain oddly silent regarding God's Lordship demands for *the rest of us,* including our bodies! This narrow spirit-alone-matters approach to salvation functionally amounts to heresy.

Most heresies throughout the centuries have centered on who Jesus is: specifically, his claim to deity (and, thus, Lordship). The first-century Gnostic heretics erroneously proclaimed that the *material* (physical matter) was inherently inferior to, and distinct from, the *spiritual.* Specifically, they taught that the body is evil, only the spirit is good. Gnosticism's destructive, heretical conclusion was that Jesus was *not* God in flesh. He was, in their view, God who only *seemed* to be flesh.[5]

A parallel heretical thought proposes that only what happens in our spirits truly matters—our bodies are not of great consequence. Many devout believers unwittingly embrace this notion, defensively arguing that *"bodily exercise profiteth little"* (1 Tim 4:8, KJV). In effect, they ignore Christ's Lordship over their bodies— until illness strikes. The English Standard Version provides a more precise translation of this important thought in 1 Timothy: *"train yourself for godliness; for while bodily training is of some value, godliness is of value in every way"* (4:7–8). Paul never demanded that believers ignore or avoid physical exercise. He clearly urged, however, that they pursue *all* of life, including exercise and food intake, through a disciplined and holistic pursuit of godliness.

5. "Gnosticism."

SETTING THE THEOLOGICAL STAGE FOR A SOLUTION

The paramount truth of Christianity is summarized in three short words: Jesus is Lord! Peter declared to Cornelius: *"You know the message God sent to the people of Israel, announcing the good news of peace through Jesus Christ, who is Lord of all"* (Acts 10:36, NIV). Similarly, Paul argued that *"what we proclaim is not ourselves, but Jesus Christ as Lord"* (2 Cor 4:5). Both of these great New Testament preachers proclaimed the same bedrock doctrine of the faith.

Christ's Lordship is, in fact, THE dominant theme of the entire New Testament (see Phil 2:9–11). His deity (and Lordship) was affirmed by the Father at his baptism (Matt 3:17) and, later, during his transfiguration (Luke 9:35). Jesus himself affirmed his Lordship: *"You call me Teacher and Lord, and you are right, for so I am"* (John 13:13). And what of us? Our holistic affirmation of Christ's Lordship—expressed through our words, actions, appetites, and lifestyle—glorifies the Father. Christ's rule over *every* aspect of our lives is our only hope for wholeness and full recovery from the Great Divide.

HEALING THE GREAT DIVIDE

Many Christians lack scriptural instruction on spiritual-physical wholeness. As a result, some easily conclude that Jesus has no great interest in their caloric intake or lifestyle. If they just avoid drugs, cigarettes, and alcohol abuse, all is *seemingly* well. Bluntly stated, this perspective is both self-deceptive and heretical because it essentially denies that Jesus is Lord of ALL!

We often laugh at gluttony displayed by others (and even in our own lives). In fact, we find creative ways of excusing ourselves for constant fleshly indulgences and sloth. Later, though, we come to Christ begging for healing when we are hurting. Even more irrational, many believers blame the Devil for their *self-inflicted* lifestyle diseases: hypertension, type 2 diabetes, gout, and many forms of heart disease. Lordship-denying, body-abusing choices have nothing to do with the Devil. They do, however, have *every-thing* to do with our functional embrace of heresy.

The word *Lord* means Lord—not medical advisor, personal trainer, or life coach! And *all* means all—not *almost* all, or *sometimes* all. I must discount large chunks of Scripture to conclude that my lifestyle, especially my exercise choices and food intake, do not matter to Christ! Paul prayed a holistic prayer for the Thessalonian believers: *"Now may the God of peace himself sanctify you completely, and may your whole spirit and soul and body be kept blameless at the coming of our Lord Jesus Christ"* (1 Thess 5:23). Obviously, all three—spirit, soul, and body—matter! Christ's *all-inclusive* Lordship directly impacts how I pursue *"godliness"* (1 Tim 4:8) and live *"to the praise of his glorious grace"* (Eph 1:6). His Lordship, thus, determines how often I put down my fork and put on my gym shoes!

Only by surrendering both spirit *and* body to his healing and holistic Lordship can we hope to recover from the Great Divide. Only his fiery touch upon a *whole* living sacrifice can reunite our fractured bodies and spirits. Freely, unreservedly, we must welcome his comprehensive claim on us as whole people. Paul challenged the Corinthians to do just this:

> Do you not know that your body is a temple of the Holy Spirit within you, whom you have from God? You are not your own, for you were bought with a price. So glorify God in your body. (1 Cor 6:19–20)

This book will inform and guide this process of honoring him with our bodies—the bodies he created. May it bear the fruit of wholeness and heresy-free living in those who honestly, freely acknowledge that Jesus Christ is Lord *of all*!

2

Living as a Grateful Steward
Harmonizing Gift and Responsibility

"Take care of your body. It's the only place you have to
live." Jim Rohn[1]

THE VAST MAJORITY OF us are born healthy.[2] That's the good news!
The bad news is we are *all* born into a fallen world. The longer
we live, the greater the impact of that fallen world, compounded
by our fallen natures. As the years pass, the impact of our often
selfish, comfort-driven choices accumulates. Even the healthier
people among us acknowledge that aging takes its toll—sometimes
painfully so. The old adage—*nobody gets out of here alive*—invariably applies, though most Christians long for a painless death or,
better still, a death-free, painless exit via the rapture of the saints
(1 Thess 4:16–18).

---

1. https://www.brainyquote.com/quotes/jim_rohn_147499.

2. I wrote this first sentence with full awareness that some infants are sick
from birth, while others become gravely ill early in life. Sick children under-
score the brokenness of our world—almost from their first breaths. I acknowledge their pain and the anguish of their caregivers.

TWO PRINCIPLES OF STEWARDSHIP

A recent Amazon search for books on stewardship yielded over 6,000 hits. Some are secular works; many are biblically focused. I feel no compulsion to compete with them![3] I highlight here only two foundational truths about biblical stewardship. First, stewards have been entrusted with *something of value*: typically this is something precious, something needing care and oversight because it is capable of being lost, stolen, damaged, or abused. Second, stewards have been entrusted with *something that is not theirs!* They may serve the Giver for a lifetime, and they may know the valued object (let's label it a "treasure" or "gift") entrusted to them like . . . . well . . . . like the back of their hand. But the treasure—their body, for example—is not truly theirs, no matter how well they know it, feed it, admire it, or smell it.

STEWARDSHIP IN BIBLICAL PERSPECTIVE

We are stewards of the bodies God has entrusted to us. Stewardship starts there—with what is nearest (often dearest) and most familiar to us. It starts with the one treasure we may be tempted to believe belongs to us: our bodies. As noted in chapter 1, Paul rebuked this temptation when reminding the Corinthians that they were neither the owners nor the masters of their bodies, for they had been "*bought with a price*" (1 Cor 6:20).

Biblically, stewards are not owners: they are simply caretakers of something belonging to Another! Accountable to the Giver for his "gift," we bear the awesome responsibility of offering our physical bodies to the Holy Spirit as his home-away-from-heaven dwelling. Wise stewards welcome him "home" by stewarding their bodies well, fully aware that those bodies are on loan from, and are entrusted to them by, God.

Most gifts we receive are *totally* free—no strings attached. In contrast, the treasured resources entrusted to stewards require

---

3. For the search results, see https://www.amazon.com/s/ref=nb_sb_noss_1?url=search-alias%3Dstripbooks&field-keywords=stewardship.

accountability: *"it is required of stewards that they be found faithful"* (1 Cor 4:2). In Matthew 25:19, all three talented[4] servants were ordered to account for what the Master had entrusted to their care. True, we normally think of God's gifts as *spiritual* in nature, such as prophecy and words of knowledge.[5] Yet *all* gifts from God must be stewarded, protected, developed, and invested in ways that create "profit" for the Giver. Warning: unprofitable servants are extremely unpopular with the Giver! Matthew 25:30 details his dreadful response to such servants!

Peter made this stewardship principle abundantly clear:

> As each has received a gift, use it to serve one another, as good stewards of God's varied grace: whoever speaks, as one who speaks oracles of God; whoever serves, as one who serves by the strength that God supplies—in order that in everything God may be glorified through Jesus Christ. (1 Pet 4:10–11)

I believe no serious damage to this passage would be inflicted if we added, "whoever has a body, as one who cares for it diligently, recognizing it is the temple of the Holy Spirit." Peter clearly believed that those who serve do so *"by the strength that God supplies"* (4:11). This phrase implies that the body receiving that strength is healthy enough, fit enough, strong enough in its own right to benefit from God's *added* strength. Make no mistake: biblical stewardship carries with it serious demands; it also generates great rewards. Divine enablement flows through those servants who are ready to do whatever their Lord requires of them . . . with bodies capable of glorifying God through Jesus Christ.

HARMONIZING THE GIFT AND ITS STEWARDSHIP RESPONSIBILITIES

God gives freely: grace, peace, mercy, his own Son. But we dare not ignore the "strings" of accountability attached to those gifts. For example, the Greatest Gift comes with strings attached: *"Whoever*

---

4. Pun intended.

5. See 1 Cor 12:8–10.

believes in him is not condemned, but whoever does not believe is condemned already, because he has not believed in the name of the only Son of God" (John 3:18). The Gift is *cost*-free, but not *obligation*-free; in the case of John 3:18, the obligation is to *"believe!"*

Similarly, God freely gave most of us healthy bodies—undeserved and unrequested. Yet he will hold us accountable for how we treat them: they are, after all, *his* temple. In great patience and mercy, God may choose to heal what *we* have damaged, abused, and neglected. Still, divine healing is not God's plan for healing self-inflicted lifestyle diseases. The ideal is God's stewards, with grateful hearts, treating their bodies as treasured gifts with amazing beauty, complexity, and power. These are gifts for which God *will* hold them accountable.

With healthy bodies, cared for and nurtured by grateful stewards, God's people can do mighty exploits. His strength and power, that powerful spiritual enablement for physical tasks, generate amazing results when allowed to flow through bodies fully devoted to his service.

To summarize, we receive gifts from him, free of our own merit, but not free of our accountability. The act of balancing these foundational aspects of life—*embracing* the free gifts and *accepting responsibility* for them—characterizes true Christian maturity. This balancing act reflects full commitment to God as both the Giver and the Lord who holds his stewards accountable (Matt 25:19). "How did you steward the body I gave you? Did you do all within your power to safeguard it, discipline it, and train it to endure hardship?"[6]

THE SPIRIT'S DWELLING PLACE

Temples of the Holy Spirit (1 Cor 6:19): what an awesome, transcendent thought this is! Grateful stewards of reasonably healthy

---

6. See 2 Tim 2:3 in the KJV.

bodies will esteem the following two pivotal statements.[7] The first of these is worded positively:

> If my body is *truly* a temple of the Holy Spirit,
> exercise becomes a language of prayer,
> cardiovascular training prolongs its service,
> strength training enhances its beauty and stamina,
> my health and wellbeing are his temple servants,
> *his* comfort and welcome remain my highest priorities.

This definition of body stewardship also impacts strongly when stated negatively (below). It identifies those actions that all body stewards must guard against:

> If my body is *truly* a temple of the Holy Spirit, I must NOT . . .
> *defile it* with spiritually offensive behaviors,
> *pollute it* with harmful or addictive substances,
> *abuse it* through unhealthy food and lack of sleep,
> *weaken it* through sloth, stress, or destructive habits,
> *threaten it* by engaging in ego-driven, risky behaviors,
> *destroy it* by any means.

May everyone who freely acknowledges both the gift—their body—and the Giver also open wide their temple's "door" to him: "Welcome, Holy Spirit! Welcome home!"

---

7. Both of these statements emerged out of monthly fasting in 2013 and 2014.

UNIT 2
Sweaty

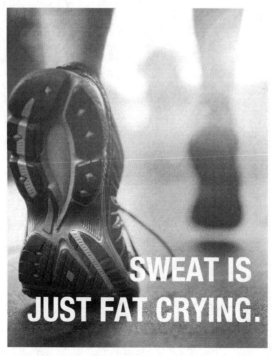

3

Created for Cardio
Minutes Matter

"God created it. Jesus died for it. The Spirit lives in it. I better take care of it." Rick Warren[1]

MADE TO MOVE

WE WERE MADE TO move. Our cardiovascular systems thrive on extended but controlled periods of serious exertion: the kind of exertion that produces sweaty t-shirts, increased heartrates, and mildly labored breathing.

The word *exertion* is not a term most of us use in daily communication. It is, nonetheless, a good word—an 8-letter word, not one of those terrible 4-letter words (e.g., *work* and *hard* and *life*)! And even if you would never actually use the word *exertion* in a real conversation, the fact[2] remains that we are at our best

---

1. http://becominghiscrown.com/2016/08/18/what-does-fitness-have-to-do-with-god/.

2. See, for example, "From Head to Toe: The Benefits of a Cardio Workout" and "4 Essential Spiritual Benefits of Physical Exercise."

mentally, physically, and (I argue) spiritually during and after a body-pushing, blood-pumping "cardio" workout. Yes, indeed, it feels really good when I *stop* at the end of my 50-minute treadmill workout. I typically step off that spiritual-discipline machine a bit shaky, a bit winded, and more than a bit sweat-soaked. But I also step off a slightly better person. I reached my goal for the day. I worked hard . . . and I survived! More importantly, I reminded my body that *it serves me*, not the other way around. And having prayed for most of those 50 minutes, I exit the gym once again offering my body as the temple of the Holy Spirit, as my Creator designed it to be.[3] After more than six years of fairly consistent cardio training,[4] I am convinced that those minutes on the treadmill, seeking to glorify Christ through that discipline, constitute serious spiritual business!

When our pulse rates are elevated for a sustained period (minutes, not seconds), followed by a gradual cool down, our entire biosystem flourishes. We thrive holistically because we generate system-wide changes[5] associated with good health. Stated differently, we are at our best when regularly engaged in some form of sustained, heart-rate-increasing activity. Researchers have clearly established that some form of cardiovascular exertion (there's that word again!) several days a week *lowers* my blood pressure, total cholesterol, and resting heartrate. It also *elevates* my HDL level (the "good" cholesterol). Finally, such exertion *increases* my metabolism, the number of new blood vessels, and overall heart health.[6]

True, cardio training is not a comfortable process. At regular intervals during workouts, my body tries to convince my mind that it is doing just fine without all that strain and fuss and (*yuk!*) sweat! My body is most uncomfortable during my occasional anaerobic[7]

---

3. See chapter 1.

4. As of August 2018, when this manuscript was completed.

5. See "Cardio Exercise Definition and Benefits."

6. See, for example, "Walk Your Way to New Blood Vessels." Note that such exertion also positively impacts mental health and immune systems.

7. "Anaerobic means 'without oxygen.' Anaerobic exercise is the type where

one-minute sprint walks, accompanied by *some* huffing and puffing—but not the kind that could blow over the homes of small piglets. Cardiovascular exercise, even at mild levels, varies between uncomfortable and occasionally painful. But we were created for this! As I argue at the start of this chapter, our bodies thrive on moderate amounts—a few hours a week—of cardio training, even though they sometimes complain loudly during the process.

Long-distance runners—those odd people who measure their workouts in miles, not feet or yards—supposedly experience a natural high or euphoric state at some point during their runs. Sedentary people (aka, "couch potatoes") often smugly observe that such runners look miserable, not even close to euphoric. But their smugness vanishes several days before their annual physicals; jokes about the thin, fit people around them fade as that appointment looms. Often overweight and under-fit, sedentary people brace for the same medical rebuke they heard last year . . . and the year before:

- "I am going to have to increase your blood pressure medication."
- "Your total cholesterol is still at a dangerous level!"
- "Your diabetes is still out of control."

If my doctor is not happy with my fitness level, general health, and artery-choking diet, *how could Jesus be?* How can I dare confess Jesus is Lord when my bathroom scale and my doctor both confess that my *body* is lord? These are questions to ponder—on the way to the gym!

MINUTES MATTER—COUNT ON IT

Minutes matter in the weird and wonderful world of cardiovascular exercise. In general, *some* exercise is better than *no* exercise.

---

you get out of breath in just a few moments, like when you lift weights for improving strength, when you sprint, or when you climb a long flight of stairs" (Weil, "Aerobic and Anaerobic Exercise: Examples and Benefits").

Some minutes are better than *no* minutes. A moderate-paced walk for twenty minutes, for example, is better than *no* minutes (i.e., *no* walk)! And, all other things being equal, forty minutes is far better than twenty minutes. Chapter 5 in this unit addresses the importance of controlling the upper limits. (A three-hour run may not, in fact, be superior to a one-hour run.) For most people,[8] "the more, the better" serves as a safe and reliable guiding principle for their cardio training.

Minutes are amazing: they exhibit an unwavering commitment, in concentrated doses, to add up to hours. And at least a couple of hours of moderate cardio exercise a week add up to improved health; those hours also result in fewer rebukes by both one's doctor and one's Lord. The American College of Sports Medicine (ACSM) offers two distinct recommendations for cardio exercise: the preferred intensity determines which recommendation to adopt.[9] At a minimum, those embracing a moderate-intensity commitment should plan to exercise for 30 (up to 60) minutes a day, five days a week: *at least* 2.5 hours total per week. In contrast, those willing (and able) to ramp up the intensity (adding speed, resistance, or incline) will benefit just as much from 20 (to 60) minutes a day, three times per week: *at least* one full hour per week of heavy breathing and sweating.

GRADUAL GAINS ARE SUSTAINABLE VICTORIES

The ACSM, cited above, urges a *"gradual progression"* [emphasis added] in a person's cardio fitness program. Status quo is not an option; we must pursue gradual fitness gains: becoming faster and stronger, possessing greater endurance. Those gains must be sustainable; and nothing threatens sustainability more than a *sudden* change in our cardio routine. If we push ourselves too hard, too quickly, for too long, we invariably threaten our motivation to put on our gym clothes again the next day, and the next, and the next.

8. Especially unfit people: unfit but medically capable of at least modest cardiovascular exertion.

9. Garber et al., "Quantity and Quality of Exercise," 1334–59.

The word *progression* in exercise is always defined with reference to the fitness triplets:

- *duration*: minutes per cardio session;
- *frequency*: number of times per week;
- *intensity*: the pace (measured by speed) of the walk, swim, run, elliptical rotations, etc.

Only a *gradual* progression in our exercise efforts allows us to maintain the motivation to continue. It also reduces the risk of injury. Athletes who sustain injuries often do so when they push themselves aggressively, dramatically exceeding their current routine. Personal bests, with reference to speed or endurance, are always set incrementally, after modest pushes.

Slow, steady, and *sane* always win the day in the world of cardio fitness. For those just starting to exercise regularly, I strongly recommend rejecting outright *any* cardio program that includes a term like *insanity, boot camp*, or *blood and guts* in its advertising. The pace and distance that pushes me today will likely feel like a modest workout three months from now. As is true of so many issues and activities in life, *gradually* ramping up the intensity of cardio exercise is the only *sustainable* strategy. A minute a day increase in duration, another tenth of a mile in distance, another 25 calories burned—all are markers of gradual (slow, steady, sane) progression. Such markers must be taken seriously and treated with respect. Minutes matter; for some, those minutes may well become a matter of life or death.

4

Goal-Focused Exercise
Track the Training

"If you want to be happy, set a goal that commands your thoughts, liberates your energy and inspires your hopes."
Andrew Carnegie[1]

TO WHERE? HOW FAST?

"Going Nowhere Slowly" was a popular television program in South Africa during the years my wife and I lived in Cape Town. It featured a group of wanderers exploring the unusual, off-the-beaten-path sights and wonders of South Africa in a decades-old Chevy Impala. Whenever they reached their destination was just fine with them, as was the duration of their stay.

Destination? Duration? Pace of the trip? None of these matter if you are going nowhere slowly! I often recall that TV show when I see people ambling down the road or sidewalk, *seemingly* for exercise. Not all activities pursued in the name of fitness qualify

---

1. https://www.success.com/18-motivational-quotes-about-successful-goal-setting/.

as meaningful cardio exercise. The facts are clear: both the *duration* and the *pace* of exercise matter. And both can (for relatively healthy people) increase over time. Yet such increases will *never* happen without clear fitness goals.

DURATION OF CARDIO EXERCISE

Let's go *somewhere*—even if on a revolving treadmill or elliptical machine (two of my favorite cardio options). A high school track or neighborhood street can work just as well.[2] Becoming fit requires only a consistent track record[3] of sustained duration. Systematically recording that duration, with either a low-tech pencil or high-tech Fitbit, enables us to repeatedly set and pursue reasonable goals for improved fitness.

Decades ago, my morbidly obese "old man" was unable (OK, *unwilling*) to sustain *any* form of cardiovascular exercise beyond 30 minutes. Gravely concerned about my sad condition, my doctor valiantly encouraged me to exercise *at least* 40 minutes per session. But those additional 10 minutes seemed totally unrealistic and unsustainable, and I told him so! At about 250 pounds then, I viewed cardiovascular exercise as an enemy, not as a friend: a demanding, painful enemy impossible to live with—*for forty minutes*! I know now that I was sabotaging my own exercise efforts by not setting modest longer-range fitness goals. This sabotage worked! Another two decades rolled past in my self-inflicted fat prison.

Imagine you have recently met a guy named Jim—perhaps the busy pastor of a growing church—who has not exercised seriously since he was in high school. But Jim has set a New Year's goal to exercise twenty minutes a day, two days a week. Under-fit and over-fed, he views those minutes in January as a serious ordeal; they constitute a major life challenge for him . . . at first. But as January turns into February and the total number of his workouts

---

2. The choice of cardio exercise, in my view, does not matter. What matters is that we find something that works, and then work it consistently, faithfully. I repeat this theme throughout Units 2 and 3.

3. Pun intended!

reach double digits, the last five minutes per day of Jim's workouts do not feel *quite* so bad. That's when he should focus on a longer-range fitness goal. Refocusing will enable him to avoid any loss of motivation to continue this strange new journey.

What longer-range goal should Jim set? I would urge him to increase the duration of *each* workout, but only by 5 percent to 10 percent a week. For example, during the first week of March he could begin stretching the duration of each cardio session to 22 minutes, then up to 23 minutes per session the second week, finally up to 25 minutes by the end of March. The level of exertion will feel about the same, but those extra five minutes per session will positively impact Jim's overall fitness—and attitude! And small successes in March will inspire new goals for April as he lengthens each workout, *systematically* and *wisely*, to 30 minutes by May 1st!

Setting realistic goals and pursuing them systematically is, in fact, foundational to Jim's future health. And he can *dramatically* stretch the duration of his new exercise program by adding a third workout to his weekly routine. Instead of limiting his cardio training to Tuesdays and Fridays, he could adopt a Monday-Wednesday-Friday (or Saturday) routine. In fact, the *frequency* during the week is just as important as the *duration* of each workout. I would say to our imaginary friend, "*Go Jim! I can't wait to see you in October!*"

I have benefited greatly by setting weekly, monthly, and even annual goals for cardio duration. My current duration goal is 2.5 hours per week: 125 hours a year (allowing two weeks missed due to travel, illness, and unforeseen obligations). At the start of every week, I remind myself: "50 minutes times 3 cardio sessions equals 2.5 hours this week!" I don't always reach that total, but the goal remains my private, voiceless "trainer" day by day as I sweat it out on the treadmill.

How high should you set your duration goal? Many experts, as noted earlier, recommend at least 40 minutes per workout, three times a week.[4] Others urge a goal of five 30-minute modest

---

4. McCoy, "Can You Lose Weight with a 40-Minute Treadmill Workout?"

cardio sessions, especially for seriously under-fit people.[5] Which is best? The goal you can achieve and sustain long term is *always* the best one! In the cardio-health domain, consistency triumphs zeal; specifically, consistency is a much wiser choice than guilt-driven bursts of unsustainable heroics.

THE PACE OF CARDIO EXERCISE

Duration is certainly goal-friendly, but what about pace? Most reasonably healthy under-fit/over-fed people are capable of walking—at least for a while—at a 3.5 mile-per-hour pace. OK, they may not see 3.5 the first few times they exercise, but they will get there if they are consistent in their efforts and patient with themselves. Novice runners can often manage 5.0 miles per hour (or faster), at least for a while. These two observations beg the question: How fast is fast enough?

As with duration, pace thrives on modest, adjustable goals. And as with duration goals, we should increase our pace goals modestly and gradually. The *immediate* goal should never push us beyond the wisdom and physical safety of a modest aerobic[6] pace. Dramatically increasing the pace of exercise usually kills preliminary fitness initiatives and motivation. When first starting a cardio-training initiative, avoid the totally winded anaerobic[7] huffing and puffing associated with the big bad wolf! Stated differently, *gradual* increases are sustainable; grandiose initial efforts pushing an under-fit body hard are generally doomed to defeat.

I have found that setting pace goals has been much easier when I am focused on the digital display of a cardio machine.

5. Miller, "7 Benefits of Doing Cardio for 30 Minutes a Day."

6. "Aerobic refers to how your body uses oxygen to sufficiently meet energy demands during exercise. . . . Aerobic exercise is any physical activity that makes you sweat, causes you to breathe harder, and gets your heart beating faster than at rest. It. . . . uses your large muscle groups, is rhythmic in nature, and can be maintained continuously for at least 10 minutes" (Ricketts, "What Is Aerobic Exercise?").

7. See chapter 3, Created for Cardio, for the definition of *anaerobic*.

Whether on a high-tech cardio machine or a lonely beach, however, we *can* control the pace of our exertion. We *can* gradually increase the pace as we increase our level of fitness. Greater fitness empowers greater effort.

My personal goal for 2018, as in recent years, is a sustained walking pace of 5.0 mph with an occasional treadmill sprint to 5.5 mph for add intensity. I have approached that sustained speed at times, but the goal continues to both elude and motivate me. Some months ago, I was able to hold a pace of 5.1 mph for about 15 minutes at a time. Ultimately, though, my heart rate exceeded my safe upper limit, and I returned to a slightly reduced pace.[8] My too-high pulse told me that my fitness level could not sustain that pace. But I am still working hard in 2018! Who knows what a fairly fit almost 70-year old guy can accomplish when buttressed by a reasonable goal?

Coping effectively with life always requires coping with change. Both our behaviors and our bodies change as we age. Flexibility and the willingness to adjust define effective living in every domain, including physical fitness. Modest goals for performance improvement, sustained over months—not just days—are foundational to health and long life. This is simply a DWI (deal with it)!

8. See chapter 5: Heart Rates Count.

5

Heart Rates Count
Boundaries, Sprints, and Water

"Let us run with endurance the race that is set before us."
Hebrews 12:1

"WE HAVE NO PULSE!" That's a statement you never want to hear
a doctor yell when you are pacing the length of a hospital waiting
room. It signals extreme danger, usually triggering a "code-blue"
emergency response by medical staff. Clearly, pulse matters—for
both the living and the dying. With a focus on the living, this chapter examines heart rate as a direct marker of physical fitness and an
indirect measure of health risks.

BOUNDARIES: PULSE IS A GOOD THING—IF NOT EXCESSIVE

Having a pulse is a good thing. Having a pulse that accurately
reflects its owner's state of exertion is a *really* good thing. Pulse
should be modestly low during times of rest, and significantly elevated during cardiovascular exercise. But how low is low? How
elevated is elevated? And how well do these numbers reflect a person's state of health?

Answers to these vital questions *always* vary with a person's age and medical history.[1] An extremely low pulse, especially for non-athletes, can be as bad as an extremely high one. In general, healthy *maximum* heart rates decline with age. A 40-year-old can max out at about 180 beats per minutes (BPM). At my current age of 69—almost 70, that rate would signal cardiovascular distress and a trip to the nearest emergency room; my maximum should never ever exceed 150 BPM.

Most of us, even during a heavy workout, never hit that upper extreme. Certainly, we should never *target* it, never view 100 percent of our age-defined maximum as a goal. We can *approach* it safely, though, by targeting 70 percent to 85 percent of our maximum BPM. Sustaining a heart rate in that range for 30 or more minutes defines effective aerobic fitness training! When relatively healthy people stress their cardiovascular systems within those boundaries, all manner of good-for-you physical changes occur. Cholesterol levels drop and metabolism rates increase. Resting heart rates and risk of stroke both decline . . . as do the numbers displayed on the bathroom scale! Great benefits accompany modest efforts in cardiovascular exercise.

What of the *minimum* side of things? How hard should our hearts work when resting? A general rule of thumb is "the lower the better:" half (or less) of an 85-percent-of-maximum BPM. True, some people have dangerously slow heart rates; those require serious medical intervention (and probably a pace-maker device). Most of us, however, should be concerned about a resting pulse that is *too high*—70 BPM (or more)—rather than one that is too low.

---

1. A widely used formula for age-defined maximum heartrates is 220 minus one's age. This formula, however, is a one-size-fits-all approach; it has *no clear research basis*. Alternative approaches, ones that reflect both age and *one's level of fitness*, are available, as discussed in the following sources:
  • Danielsson, "How to Calculate Your Heart Rate!"
  • "How to Calculate Target Heart Rate Zone?"
  • "Maximum Heart Rate Formula."
  • Robergs and Landwehr, "The Surprising History of the HRmax=220-age Equation," 1–10.

OUR ADAPTABLE BODIES

Our bodies have an amazing ability to adapt to what we routinely do to them. The range of adaptation is, however, not infinite: I will never have the resting pulse of a 30-year-old marathon winner! Within limits, I (that is, my body) will adapt to my cardio exercise regimen: one of the joyous-painful discoveries I have made on the treadmill. A given pace—4.7 miles per hour (mph), for example—that pushed my heart rate to 85 percent of my maximum in February may not even raise it to 80 percent a few months later. This awesome, rewarding adaptation, called *fitness*, is clearly evidenced on my treadmill's digital display. The higher my fitness level, the lower my pulse—both during and between cardio sessions.

Our ability to adapt to self-imposed levels of exertion is both predictable and somewhat frustrating. For example, if I maintain a 4.7 mph pace during my 50-minute aerobic-pace walk, my fitness level will slowly decline over time. And as I adapt, my heart rate will decrease *slightly*, my sweat-soaked t-shirt notwithstanding. Eventually, this persistent adaptation downward permits the sneaky return of bad-for-me things like elevated LDL cholesterol levels.

As my heart rate falls below my age-defined 85-percent goal, I must make a key decision. I need to increase the sustained speed of my walk to 4.8 mph, for example, or find another way (such as brief anaerobic sprints) to safely challenge my body's persistent adaptation! Both are reasonable options, ones that can be used in tandem. This aerobic-anaerobic mix, discussed in the following section, is an ideal strategy for increasing fitness levels.

SPRINTS: FROM AEROBIC TO ANAEROBIC, AND BACK AGAIN

Watching world-class sprinters burn up a 100-meter track is exhilarating. In less time than it takes to walk to the fridge (again) for a snack, their race is over. These amazing speedsters, including short-distance hurdlers, generate great speed and power for short distances: 200 meters or less. Their bursts of speed are clearly anaerobic,[2] leaving them slightly winded at the finish line despite intense, year-round training. That is the nature of anaerobic cardio training. And that is why Usain Bolt and other speedsters do not compete in 5,000 meter races. Their sprint-based training, heavily into the anaerobic zone, could not prepare them for races requiring sustained aerobic effort.

Anaerobic exercise requires high-intensity effort that exceeds the body's capacity for sustained muscle performance. Try sprinting as fast as you can go for 150 yards. Your body will start screaming for oxygen before you finish, leaving you sucking air and unable to talk normally . . . for a while. If you immediately start walking at a decent aerobic pace, your breathing will return to a comfortable rate. The sooner this happens, the better your fitness level.

Health and fitness promoters generally agree that modest, aerobic-pace distance training combined with brief almost-all-out (anaerobic-pace) sprinting generate maximum increases in cardiovascular health. The key to this mix is returning to the slower aerobic pace for an extended time immediately *after* the brief anaerobic sprint. As breathing returns to an exercise-normal level and heart rate slows some, powerful changes impact the body:

- Heart is stronger;
- Lungs increase their capacity;
- Oxygen level in the body increases;
- Pulse slows;
- You feel great, thankful that the anaerobic sprint is over.

Returning now to my treadmill decision, what do I do when my heart rate is no longer challenged by 4.8 mph? I "sprint," briefly, by bumping the speed up by 0.5 to 5.3 mph. I hold it there for 45 to 60 seconds, then slow to 4.9 (not 4.8) mph. My breathing returns fairly quickly to treadmill normal and my legs morph from jelly back into muscle. A few minutes later, 4.9 feels about like 4.8 did

2. See footnote 7 in chapter 3. See also "Aerobic vs. Anaerobic: What's Best for Weight Loss?"

before the sprint! That is *the* most amazing thing about adding one or two short-duration sprints to a 50-minute aerobic session! And I become slightly more fit in the process.

WATER IS OUR FRIEND

A year or so into my serious weight loss, I discovered that water intake dramatically lowers my heart rate. After about twenty minutes of walking, my heart rate relentlessly edges upward. A *too*-high pulse is almost certain, especially if I have included a brief treadmill sprint at about the ten-minute mark.

Prior to discovering the power of water, I was forced to either slow down or briefly step off the belt. I still do both, but I can delay these strategies by first downing some water. The first drink lowers my heart rate about ten beats per minute, taking me back under my self-imposed maximum. Amazing!

After some minutes of water-empowered brisk walking, my heart rate again starts creeping upward. I control it with another long gulp or two, continuing this process throughout the rest of my cardio session. Admittedly water offers diminishing returns: after 35 minutes or so, it no longer significantly impacts my heart-rate. Still, water remains my cardio friend because it extends the pace and duration of my workouts. I'll drink to that!

6

Consistency and Moderation
Foundations of Lasting Fitness

"Moderation in all things, especially moderation." Ralph
Waldo Emerson[1]

RESOLUTIONS: NEW YEAR VS. OLD YEAR

ONE OF THE GREATEST abuses of tempt-able consumers occurs
each January. Merchants begin advertising a variety of fitness
equipment, targeting millions of turkey-stuffed and over-*stuff*-
ed[2] folk desperate for a major change in their lives. Year after
year, consumers eagerly embrace the delusional hope embedded
in the phrase "New Year's Resolutions." Gym memberships are
half-off, but "for a limited time only." Creative exercise gizmos
line the "seasonal" aisles in stores, replacing the unsold Christmas
tinsel. Wondrous new diets are enthusiastically promoted by actors wearing white coats and stethoscopes. Advertisers love this

1. https://www.goodreads.com/quotes/86634-moderation-in-all-things-
especially-moderation.
2. "Stuff" in this usage refers to Christmas gifts in excessive supply.

immune-to-reality season almost as much as Christmas itself. What little cash remains after the holidays again becomes easy picking from the frustrated masses.

Year after year, millions sadly observe January's bold resolutions retreat before February's discouraging reality. The sincerest promises made to self and others will likely be broken . . . again! Enticed by images of people who lost 40 pounds doing this or using that, millions set themselves up for repeated defeat by embracing immodest expenditures and unsustainable efforts. January's expensive new exercise equipment is eventually dragged to the over-*stuff*-ed garage to await April's garage sale, at 75-percent discount!

But people *can* change; people *do* change—sometimes permanently so! Lasting fitness changes will, however, forever elude and frustrate those who are unwilling to pursue consistency and true lifestyle adjustments in small, incremental steps. For well over forty years, I was morbidly obese and morbidly miserable. I daily carried the burden of 60 to 80 fat pounds wherever I went. From third grade onward, I wore Husky Boy jeans outside and self-defeat inside. As an adult, *every* day, *multiple times a day*, I dreamed of—longed for—dramatic, lasting weight loss. Yet my New Year's "resolutions" eventually became little more than fuzzy wishes. I was trapped in a lifestyle that glorified self-indulgence and comfort eating—until that one November day!

TAPPING THE POWER OF HABIT STRENGTH

On November 30, 2011, a wild idea gripped me: "I can lose a kilo [2.2 pounds] a week for 30 weeks, as a 40th wedding anniversary gift to Rosie." The next day, thirty weeks prior to our anniversary, I began to (1) eat two meals a day (brunch and dinner), (2) resist the tempting power of food, (3) weigh myself multiple times a day, and (4) apply sustained, goal-focused energy to creating this "gift" for my wife. Thus began my unplanned experimentation with *Old Year's* resolutions, illustrated below. The changes I created during these thirty weeks also provided the foundations of the "diet"—the ELF[3] diet—that transformed my life!

My weight-loss success during the following sixteen months convinced me that resolutions to change our lives work best when we are not recovering from holiday self-abuse. The relatively small changes we make, like eating two modest meals a day—and only when hungry,[4] empower the growth of positive habits. It is our *habit strength*, not our best intentions, that sustains us when we are tempted by food. Consistent positive changes in how we eat, exercise, think, and live build the habits that *keep us going* (to the gym) and *on the straight and narrow* (to reasonable goal achievement). This explains the amazing power of an Old Year's resolution. My first 21 days of focused, documented weight loss in December 2011—about 7 pounds—created the habit strength I needed to get through the 2011 Christmas season *without weight gain*! I cannot remember a prior Christmas season in which I did not gain weight during that "most wonderful time of the year!"

CONSISTENT FITNESS TRAINING

Lifestyles matter. Fitness matters. Self-discipline matters. What we *do* consistently models clearly who we *are* internally. Christ-followers are called to strive for consistency in their walk with the Master (Matt 25:21; Heb 10:39). We are not permitted to judge another's spiritual journey (Matt 7:1). Still, many Christians openly display abundant waist-line evidence of spiritual dysfunction. How can they thrive spiritually when so unfit physically? Philosopher Ludwig Wittgenstein[5] argued that "the human body is the best picture of the human soul."

We need consistency as much as we need variety, perhaps more so. Many well-intended fitness resolutions fail early on for lack of consistency and the habit-strength that consistency births.

---

3. Eat Less Food. See appendix C for the details about the ELF "diet" that became, for me, a sustainable new approach to eating.

4. See unit 4: "Sometimes Hungry."

5. http://izquotes.com/quote/200890.

Consistent training demands the same *number of days* (five to six), week after week, month after month—at the same *time of day* (whenever possible). Some people prefer an early-morning workout, others favor an after-work routine. Researchers actively debate the physiological advantages of morning versus evening exercise. As noted in chapter 4,[6] I advocate a practical choice: find something that works and *work it!* Day after day, work it. Even when you do not feel energetic or emotionally "up," *show up*—same time, same place—and do *at least some* of that day's normal workout. Consistency *always* trumps intentions, resolutions, excuses, and heroic initial efforts!

MODERATION IS A VIRTUE

Moderation—avoiding lifestyle extremes while remaining actively committed to life—has long been considered a Christian virtue. Pascal[7] warned, "to go beyond the bounds of moderation is to outrage humanity. The greatness of the human soul is shown by knowing how to keep within proper bounds." Even great devotion to Christ does not eliminate the need for virtuous avoidance of excesses in other arenas of life, including cardiovascular exercise and strength training. The kind of physical fitness that glorifies Christ *never* demands extremes or obsessions. Our obsessions must remain focused on him alone.

MODERATION IN FITNESS TRAINING

How much is enough? How fast is fast enough? How long is long enough? In earlier years (outside the gym), I embraced the philosophy that anything worth doing is worth *over*-doing! While this thought still pulls on me in some areas of work and productivity, I have not allowed it to join me in the gym. More is not *always* better!

6. See footnote 2 in chapter 4.

7. http://izquotes.com/quote/375840.

As I noted in chapter 4,[8] a few decades ago my doctor sternly admonished me to spend at least 40 minutes, three times a week, in sustained cardio exercise. Though I foolishly rejected his counsel then, I know now he was right. Forty minutes, three times a week, is a useful initial goal for improving cardiovascular fitness. Some experts advocate fewer minutes of sustained cardio exertion on a five-to-seven-days-a-week schedule.[9] Which approach is best? My recommendation, stated above, is to find a weekly exercise pattern that works . . . and work it consistently.

I value both strength[10] and cardio training. Therefore, I limit my cardio training to three every-other-day sessions a week. At the risk of overstating the obvious, the math is simple: my weekly goal of 2.5 hours of cardio training requires completion of three 50-minute cardio sessions.

MODERATION VS ALL THINGS "EXTREME"

Some Christians eagerly endure the physical demands of marathon races or other extreme endurance competitions. They often testify that their commitment to the training required for such events has transformed their lives. Dramatic weight loss and increased physical fitness (and stamina) are, unquestionably, associated with the demanding training for such events.

I do not question the transforming nature of extreme competitions. My concern centers on the extent to which the lives of these competitors are dominated by their training—to say nothing of the expense and life interruptions created by the travel to such events. Weeks of grueling training over extreme distances demand the investment of hundreds of hours. Those hours must be carved out of other pursuits, taking precious time from family, career, and even devotional growth.

---

8. See the section in chapter 4 entitled "Duration of Cardio Exercise."

9. See, for example, "Cardiovascular Exercise & Weight Loss."

10. See chapter 7.

Efforts to prepare a welcoming temple for the Holy Spirit's dwelling do not require heroics or extreme fitness. In all domains of life, except in reference to loving Jesus, moderation is the key to success. Embrace moderation as a lifestyle. Run with it . . . or walk with it, as your fitness level allows!

UNIT 3

Sore

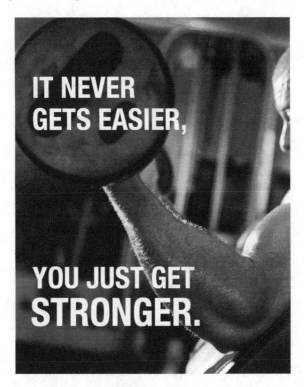

7

Strength

Foundation of Spiritual and Physical Health

"They who wait for the Lord shall renew their strength; they shall mount up with wings like eagles; they shall run and not be weary; they shall walk and not faint." Isaiah 40:31

WE'VE ALL SEEN IMAGES of body builders, with muscles bulging in places most of us didn't know humans have places. Their body fat reduced to amazingly (dangerously?) low levels, these dedicated men and women strut their near-buff stuff before admiring crowds and critical judges. The reaction of many Christians to bodybuilders ranges from admiration, to confusion, to disgust. The disgust reaction is usually accompanied by biblical warnings about placing *"confidence in the flesh"* (Phil 3:3), loving *"the flesh"* (Jude 23), and embracing the *"pride of life"* (1 John 2:16). Is it possible to pursue stronger muscles without embracing "the flesh"? Can I rejoice in the number of pushups I can do without sinful boasting about the arms that powered them? These honest questions need honest answers—answers that are found in Scripture.

STRENGTH IS A GODLY CHARACTERISTIC

God is strong! Strength is a key aspect of his nature. Through the prophets, God often describes himself as a powerful deliverer: freeing and protecting those he loves by his *"right hand"* and his *"holy arm"* (Ps 98:1). Similarly, Isaiah proclaimed *"the Lord has bared his holy arm"* before all the nations (Isa 52:10). Obviously, God is not muscle-bound like bodybuilders; still, he used the terms *"strength"* and *"powerful arm"* to describe himself (Jer 27:5, NLT). Not surprisingly, he uses the same terms to describe those he blesses:

- The psalmist declared, *"Awesome is God from his sanctuary . . . he is the one who gives power and strength to his people"* (Ps 68:35; see also Ps 29:11);

- Isaiah prophesied that God would give *"power to the faint, and to him who has no might he increases strength"* (40:29);

- Twice in one chapter, God commanded Joshua as Israel's new leader to *"be strong and courageous"* (Josh 1:6, 9). Israel echoed God's repeated command in the same chapter as they swore allegiance to Joshua as their new leader (Josh 1:18). This was an intense command, one that Joshua later passed on to Israel's army (Josh 10:25).

Concluding that such verses speak only of inner spiritual strength inflicts interpretive damage on their content; God longs to see his children walking in both spiritual *and* physical strength. The battles Joshua would soon fight required holistic strength and stamina.

Consider Caleb, Joshua's fellow spy (Num 13) and faith-filled friend, as he boldly requested the right to take on the dreaded Anakim:

> And now, behold, I am this day eighty-five years old. I am still as strong today as I was in the day that Moses sent me; my strength now is as my strength was then, for war and for going and coming. So now give me this hill country of which the Lord spoke on that day, for you heard on that day how the Anakim were there, with great fortified cities.

*It may be that the Lord will be with me, and I shall drive
them out just as the Lord said.* (Josh 14:10–12)

It was the Anakim—giants in the land of Promise—who
caused the ten fearful, faithless spies to contaminate the faith and
confidence of God's people (Num 13:31–33). Yet this 85-year-old
man was boldly declaring that his strength had not abated: his
courage, faith, *and* arms were as strong and eager for battle as
they had been four decades earlier! He was ready to take on the
giants who indirectly caused him to waste forty years of his life
wandering through the wilderness, watching his faithless friends
die one by one. As I approach my 70th birthday, I choose strong
and ready-to-fight Caleb as a key role model in my active pursuit
(my *"going and coming"*: Josh 14:11) of strength and fitness.

STRENGTH IS ESSENTIAL
TO SKELETAL HEALTH AND GENERAL VITALITY

New exercise gizmos never excite me, especially those displayed by
sweaty, beautiful actors claiming you never need to enter another
gym. (I need a gym and am not seeking ways to avoid entering
mine!) What *does* hold my attention, however, is the presenters'
consistent script: this amazing new product will "strengthen your
core"—while miraculously slimming and trimming your woefully
out-of-shape body.

Core strength is, in fact, *profoundly* important: far more so
than slimming and trimming your body. The muscles in your
abdomen, back, and sides literally hold you together. Poor core
strength almost guarantees that you will NOT thrive physically.
Underdeveloped, rarely-exercised core muscles cause people to
fall apart—painfully so in areas involving their skeletal system.
Back pain, especially in the lower back, serves as a debilitating signal that core muscles are not up to the task of holding the lumbar
vertebrae in place. And chronic low back pain usually manifests
elsewhere in the spine, including headache-inducing neck pain.
A person with strong core muscles may occasionally struggle with

back pain, but will generally recover faster and have far fewer "bad days" than his or her weaker neighbor.

Strengthening core muscles, for most of us, has nothing to do with developing a "six pack" of abdominal muscles. The issue is not how "hot" or "buff" we look, it's whether we can stand up easily— whether we can function without recurring headaches or general weakness in everyday activities. Most of our full-body movements are powered by core muscles, supplemented by the strength in our legs and arms. This means that weak core muscles will negatively impact almost *everything* we do in life, from carrying groceries in from the car to rearranging the furniture in the living room. We must develop strong core muscles to enjoy mobility, vitality, and pain-free active living!

STRENGTH IS ESSENTIAL FOR FAT REDUCTION

A pound of fat and a pound of muscle weigh the same . . . obviously! However, the pound of muscle burns *far more* calories (7 to 10 a day) than does the pound of fat (2 to 3 a day).[1] This is why strong, muscular people typically have high basal metabolic rates (BMRs): they burn a significantly high number of calories each day, even when resting! This is almost like cheating! More muscle means less fat, largely because well-developed muscles burn (metabolize) more available calories before the body can store them as fat.[2]

Look again at this section's heading: it states "fat reduction," not "weight reduction." The fact that muscle is somewhat heavier than fat suggests that strength training may actually increase (somewhat) the numbers on the scale, at least initially. As muscles grow and fat shrinks, those addicted to their scale digital displays may become discouraged. But we must never sacrifice muscle development for some arbitrarily selected ideal weight. We would be

1. Mack, "Is It a Myth that Muscle Burns More Calories than Fat?" For additional details, see Magee, "8 Ways to Burn Calories and Fight Fat."
2. "Does Building Muscle Burn Fat, Calories & Increase Metabolism?"

far wiser to adopt some measure of ideal *strength*, then commit to the weekly training needed to achieve that ideal.

Strength training becomes especially important as we grow older, when our BMRs tend to drop as both muscle strength *and* physical activity in general decline. The most effective way to *slow*, not stop, this decline is a moderate strength-training routine two to three days a week.[3] Strengthening the largest muscle groups— thighs, abdomen, back, and chest—yields the most effective fat-burning results.[4]

Actively pursuing greater physical strength requires intentional, challenging, often painful effort. This is especially true as we age. Even so, through a moderate pursuit of strength training, we can seek the blessing Moses bestowed upon the tribe of Asher: *"as your days, so shall your strength be"* (Deut 33:25).

---

3. As detailed in chapter 8 and in appendix A, my own strength-training routine includes two days of fairly intense weight lifting and a third day ("weightless Wednesday") of planking and other forms of resistance training using my own body weight.

4. Adapted from Magee (cited above).

8

Sore Muscles

Harmless but Not Painless

"The pain you feel today is the strength you feel tomorrow." Author Unknown

MUSCLES GET SORE WHEN PUSHED HARD: THAT'S A DWI

ONE OF THE SOMETIMES painful principles of life, "use it or lose it," affects us all. This principle impacts us relentlessly as we grow older. Compare the then-and-now photos of former professional athletes. Or ask the person with a shoulder injury about the pain involved in recovering from a "frozen" shoulder. Any joint immobilized for weeks will require wrenching rehab sessions. Without rehab, the joint will continue to deteriorate from lack of full, natural use.

Our musculature demonstrates a unique equivalent of this use-it-or-lose-it principle: "building strength demands pain." OK, it's not stated in exactly those terms in the fitness literature. (Actually, I just made it up!) But the principle is valid, nonetheless! Muscles become sore when they are pushed hard—when we demand more effort from them than they are normally required to produce. Beginning weight lifters are tempted to think they have pulled or torn something. Veteran lifters, in contrast, know their muscles ache after a harder-than-normal session. Even when those veteran lifters add a new lift or two, their newly targeted muscles will always complain—loudly!

My own strength-training program illustrates this principle of muscle use. I typically do two rounds (*sets*) of each of my strength-training exercises. If I add a third set on a Monday, my suddenly sore muscles will complain until at least Wednesday! *Building strength demands pain!*

So, you begin a brand new strength-training effort—maybe as an "old year[1] resolution." Or you decide to "up your game," intensifying your existing training by (1) adding new lifts, (2) lifting heavier weights than you have been using, or (3) increasing the number of reps per set.[2] You begin the day with enthusiasm, yet end the day feeling shaky and deeply fatigued. You wake up the next day feeling like a small truck hit you during the night. You hurt all over! Sore and tired, you are obsessed with the thought of taking a "sick day" at work. What will you do? What *will* you do? Never return to the gym again? Demand a refund for that year-long membership?

In your pain, you face a DWI (deal with it) situation! Likely you have not torn, ripped, broken, or cracked anything. You have simply lifted weights . . . hard . . . and it hurts! Instead of quitting, you deal with the pain by going back to the gym the next day for a modest-intensity *cardio* workout. And the following day, you train those use-them-or-lose-them muscles . . . *again!* That may not be your best ever strength-training workout, but you show up! And you lift as best you can. The weights should be lighter than normal, but you show up! By working through the pain and soreness, you grow a bit stronger. And stronger (in moderation) is good—*very* good!

---

1. See "Tapping the Power of Habit Strength" in chapter 6.
2. See chapter 9 for details.

BEWARE THE THIRD DAY

It is one of the odd realities of life for those gaining strength and building muscle. The day after a heavy workout may certainly be uncomfortable: sore, stiff muscles complicate daily activities. For some odd reason, however, the *next* day (the day *after* tomorrow) is actually the worse: this is yet another DWI situation! This phenomenon actually has a name: Delayed Onset Muscle Soreness[3] (DOMS). Thanks to DOMS, those tired, stressed muscles that got you through Monday's heavy workout are crying *loudly* on Wednesday. That's the *bad* news, and it is news you cannot ignore.

What about the *good* news? The day after tomorrow will eventually end. The other good news is that lifting that day will substantially *reduce* that pain, not make it worse. Two tried-and-true steps, suggested above, can help you overcome DOMS:

1. Complete a medium-intensity *cardio* workout on Tuesday (after Monday's heavy lifting), warming up slowly before starting. The increased circulation from the cardio workout will help those strained muscles (with thousands of micro-tears in the fibers) to heal faster.

2. Complete your normal *strength-training* workout on Wednesday, but with somewhat lighter weights. As during step 1, warm up slowly! Start your lifting routine after extensive slow, gentle stretching movements. Push your body, gently!

Listen to your body, but do not let it control you. God gave you a strong body to serve you . . . and him. You do not live to serve your body; it *must* be the other way round!

FREE WEIGHTS VS. MACHINE WEIGHTS?

Few topics in the strength-training literature generate more debate than whether free weights (e.g., dumb bells) or machine weights

---

3. Sarnataro, "Sore Muscles? Don't Stop Exercising."

(e.g., universal machines) are best.[4] Many professional trainers advocate using both types, but favor free weights—at least this is my impression. Which is better? My guarded response is, "the one that works best for you, given your age, health history, life circumstances, and available equipment."

Let's suppose you have never seriously lifted weights, but have access to a well-equipped gym and can afford to hire a professional trainer for *at least* ten training sessions. Hire the trainer[5] and follow his or her advice throughout those first training sessions. Do NOT, however, allow your new trainer to push you hard at first; you should be honest with your new trainer about this issue before you enter the weight room. You are not auditioning for The Biggest Looser! Your underdeveloped muscles, knowledge, and attitude all need time to adjust. You need a trainer who will encourage your honest effort, but will also allow you to *ease into* serious strength training.[6] One set of eight reps (or so) per lift will work wonders, stopping *before* you reach total muscle fatigue. The front end of a serious strength-training commitment is not the time for heroics.

If you have access to a gym, but cannot afford a trainer, I urge you start with machine weights. Fewer things can go wrong, and injuries are less likely. Faster weight adjustments—going heavier or lighter—are possible on a machine. View some helpful YouTube videos on machine-based workouts, then design your own training regimen. A few such videos are listed at the end of this chapter.

If you are access-less (no gym and no trainer), check out the YouTube videos (in the following section) for exercises you can do

---

4. See, for example, "Free Weights vs. Machines: Which Is Better?"

5. First, confirm with your medical provider that you can safely pursue active fitness training.

6. Many years ago while home from Africa for a year, I joined a gym. My new membership included an hour of free individual training. My trainer was terrible: he pushed me to max out my reps on multiple lifts. Afterward, I hurt so badly I could not sleep for days without medication. Some "trainers" have no compassion or understanding of how the muscles and the mind of an unfit person work. *Avoid such trainers, even if their services are technically free.*

using resistance bands[7] and your own body resistance.[8] If possible, hire a trainer for a limited number of sessions to show you some serious no-weights exercises. Or ask a veteran strength-training friend to help you get started.

In my own strength-training program, I use both: free weights for a limited number of exercises, and machine weights for the rest of my heavier lifting.[9] This is both a personal preference and an adaptation to the fact that I lift alone. Honestly, the thought of pushing through that last bench-press rep with a heavily loaded free-weight barbell and no "spotter" to help me (just in case) is terrifying. A seated chest-press machine is far less threatening: using it, I have no fear of dropping 200 pounds on my throat! Greater, faster gains in muscle development are possible with free weights (and a trainer). I have simply chosen a safer (machine weights) and less expensive (no trainer) route to strength training. As is true of cardio training, my advice is always to find something that works . . . *and work it!*

YOUTUBE VIDEOS OF INTEREST

- Free weights vs. machines: https://youtu.be/nUeQUyCWUPg
- Machine weight lifts—for beginners (female): https://youtu.be/m7yWc67-le8
- Machine weight lifts—for beginners (male): https://youtu.be/cqXMbW4rMIo
- Resistance bands (female): https://youtu.be/WIKrcoO86h4
- Resistance bands (male): https://youtu.be/mvosEeAUSTY
- Bodyweight exercises—beginners (female): https://youtu.be/5Om6M8elJtg

7. See Elkaim, "This Resistance Band Workout Routine Will Get You Toned."

8. See, for example, "5 Health Benefits of Doing Plank Exercise."

9. See appendix A for details about my strength-training program.

- Bodyweight exercises—beginners (male): https://youtu.be/L77b57erQ4M

- Bodyweight exercises—advanced training (male): https://youtu.be/ZA8GzhFh_CQ

9

Asking Questions
A Modest Pursuit of Personal Best

"Constantly think about how you could be doing things
better. Keep questioning yourself." Elon Musk[1]

A LINK EXISTS BETWEEN asking questions and strength training...
really! The two may seem totally unrelated. We ask questions
when we don't know, when we are uncertain or confused—not
when pumping iron. Mostly, we ask questions when we are *igno-
rant*—and therein lies the intentional connection. For well over
three hundred weeks[2] now, I have worked to become stronger on
Mondays, Wednesdays, and Fridays; these are days I enter the gym
feeling my ignorance. What weight can I handle today? How many
pushups this time? Inquiring minds want to know! (Well, at least
one mind does!)

1. http://www.supplychaintoday.com/elon-musk-quotes/.
2. As of the completion of this manuscript: August 2018.

ASKING QUESTIONS ABOUT SETS AND REPS

Technically the words *sets* and *reps* (repetitions) are useful four-letter words. A set is simply a group of reps—perhaps eight to ten (8–10) non-stop reps of a given lift (for example, bicep curls). Normally I finish one set, rest briefly,[3] then complete another. That second set works best under one of two conditions that I control. I sometimes leave the amount of weight unchanged, expecting fewer reps—maybe five to seven (5–7) during the second set. On other lifts, I reduce the amount of weight *slightly*, then push hard to complete the same number of reps as in the first set.

In *every* set, I strive to max out my lifting capacity: as many reps as my tiring muscles can produce while approaching anaerobic fatigue.[4] If the initial weight is too light, I will know it after only one or two reps. I stop, set the weight heavier, then resume the effort. As suggested above, I want to produce only eight to ten (8–10) maxed-out reps per set[5]; completing the last rep in each set should always be impossible. Muscle exhaustion, though painful, is my friend: maximum effort yields measurable gains.

How many reps can I complete during a given set? Can I get one more than last time . . . *just one more?* Is it time to increase the weight for both sets . . . *just a little heavier?* What is my limit today? These are among the "great questions" of my strength-training life. Audaciously asking questions when starting each set reminds me that I do not know my body's true capacity. Are more gains possible? Have I reached my limit? I am strongly motivated to know.

I'm never sure exactly how many reps I can do until I reach exhaustion, with muscles briefly depleted. But asking the key

3. Or I shift to another lift that targets a different muscle group, alternating between the two lifts to finish two sets with each.

4. I don't do this until I have actively trained for a few weeks to ensure my muscles are ready for such effort.

5. Three basic repetition strategies are (1) building muscle strength [up to 6 reps], (2) building muscle mass [ideally 8 to 10 reps], and (3) building muscle endurance [15+ reps]. I have chosen strategy 2—muscle mass—as a mid-point strategy. See the interesting YouTube video on this topic at https://www.youtube.com/watch?v=1bP5AvsRex4.

questions at the start of (and even during) a set *eventually* empowers me to lift heavier weights and become *just a bit* stronger in the process.

ASKING QUESTIONS ABOUT PACE

The pace of a strength-training session is determined by the amount of recovery time between sets and between lifts. The shorter the wait time, the more intense the workout, since muscles must produce more work in a shorter time.

What pace will I set today? The answer to this key question should impact my entire workout. Honestly, that answer is usually influenced by my out-of-gym schedule. At other times, it reflects a pre-workout decision to push myself harder for several sessions, to see what gains I make during that period. On days I do not ask the pace question, I tend to settle into a relatively comfortable rhythm that does not truly max out my potential.

My objective when entering the gym is to *leave* the gym—satisfied, sweaty, tired, and *just a tiny bit* stronger—but still, to leave! A fast-paced workout gets me out of the gym and back to real life much sooner than slowly recovering between sets and between lifts. My life largely exists *outside* the gym, not *in* it. Work, ministry, and family must all be set aside while I am pumping iron. I never want to extend a strength-training session longer than is needed to accomplish my modest strength-training goals.

ASKING QUESTIONS OF GRAVITY

Most of the questions I ask in the gym are me-focused. But I recently discovered the power of asking *gravity* a few questions, too! When preparing to start a set of pushups, I often ask the floor (aka, *gravity*) a question: "Can you stop *these* arms? Can you keep me from getting 50 pushups *this* set?" In fact, I had just asked the floor these questions when I achieved my current personal best!

I pose similar questions to the weight machines I use. On the leg-curl machine, I typically ask, "Can you stop *these* legs from getting 12 reps this set?" These, too, are ultimately gravity-focused questions. The answers I get (through my performance) to these questions sometimes happily surprise me!

When questioning gravity, I usually set a performance goal for a particular exercise. Goal-setting is a powerful way of fighting my body's tendency to acclimate or adjust to my repeated demands on it. Ask questions! Set goals! Track the gains!

ASKING QUESTIONS ABOUT ROUTINE

We are all creatures of habit; creating routines simplifies the process of getting through the day. A memorized routine eliminates time-wasting decisions about what to do next. With our routines riveted to the walls of our brains, we know exactly what to do next. Ignoring the bewildering array of free weights and weight machines around us, we can *routinely* move directly to the next lift: crunches to squats to "lat"[6] row machine, and so forth. Months in the gym generate useful, time-saving routines that pull us forward through our workouts. Habit-fueled routines guide and motivate serious strength-training efforts.

Occasionally stopping to ask a question or two about our gym routine keeps us open to new possibilities, and to more efficient use of time and equipment. A routine is a servant, not a master; it exists (through extensive experience) only to simplify our lives and save us time. Adding a new lift after watching others doing it might improve our overall workout: "Should I do that lift, too?" Deleting a lift that no longer challenges us is a wise routine-modifying decision: "Is this lift really helping me?" No routine should ever become question-proof or set in stone!

6. "Latissimus Dorsi."

ASKING QUESTIONS ABOUT MOTIVES

As suggested above, the gym exists to serve me, not to dominate my life. Watching my personal best on a particular lift s-l-o-w-l-y increasing over a few months is deeply rewarding. And the behaviors generating rewarding experiences are usually repeated: satisfying accomplishments become addictive. Therein lies the temptation of prolonged strength-training workouts: the gym can tempt me to stay longer and lift harder. It can seduce me into adding new lifts and more sets to an already-heavy routine. Minutes can easily become hours. Mirrors can easily become temples of self-worship. These are real temptations for serious lifters!

"Aren't you too old to be doing this?" My colleague's question caught me off guard. Why *am* I inflicting these physical challenges on my aging body? Am I wanting to just look "buff" as an almost 70-year old? Ridiculous! Do I want to discover my real limits? Yes! Am I working hard to prepare a strong, fit body as a temple for the Holy Spirit? Oh, *yes*! May this final goal remain my deepest motivation!

I do not ask the motive question every workout or even every month, but I do ask it—especially during my out-of-gym reflection and prayer. The gym constitutes one strategy for presenting my body *"as a living sacrifice"* to God (Rom 12:1)[7] as I strive to live (holistically, honestly, physically) *"to the praise of his glory"* (Eph 1:12).

7. See chapter 16.

UNIT 4
Sometimes Hungry

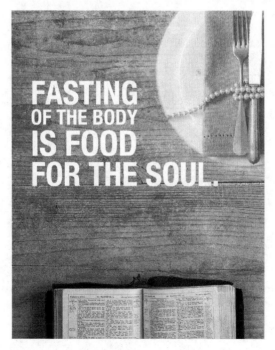

10

Fasting and the Christian Life
Mastering Hunger and Cravings

> "Learn to have restraint in food; by temperance, you will bring health and strength to the body and vigor to the mind, so needed for the work of salvation." Saint Ignatius Brianchaninov[1]

WHAT IS FASTING?

FASTING IS DELIBERATELY ABSTAINING from something important—typically food, in one form or another—for a given time period. A true fast is always a self-denying choice, with food purposefully left in the fridge, in sharp contrast to running out of food and having nothing to eat. And fasting almost always pursues some spiritual or physical benefit (perhaps both).

Fasts range from abstaining from selected food items during liturgical fasting periods (especially the Lenten fast before Easter) to water-only fasts. The "Daniel fast" (see Dan 1:12), consisting of veggies and water, is highly valued by many Christians, especially

1. http://orthochristian.com/50335.html.

those not eager to attempt the water-only "Jesus fast" (see Matt 4:1–2). Daniel's fast, in fact, closely resembles the liturgical fasts still faithfully embraced by a billion Christians worldwide.

During the forty days of Lent (Great Lent[2]), millions of the faithful also "give up" targeted sources of pleasure or entertainment: movies, social media, or time-consuming hobbies. Such religiously inspired acts clearly express a beneficial form of self-denial. Still, they do not constitute *fasting* as used in this unit.

WHY DO PEOPLE FAST?

Non-Christian motives for fasting vary widely, from eastern-religion asceticism to humanistic, self-centered fasts for various physical, mental, and "spiritual" benefits.[3] Secular fasting gurus abound, promoting their latest bestselling books on National Public Radio—books that cost much more than a combo meal at your favorite fast-food restaurant. Running contrary to our society's incessant addiction to *more*, a growing number of non-religious people are now embracing *less*!

As defined in this unit, all fast-ers abstain from some or all food for a greater good. For Christians, that greater good centers on answered prayers, and becoming more like Christ, more sensitive to God at work in their lives, and more victorious in their daily living. Many Christians also pursue the secondary motive of becoming healthier people. Physical health and spiritual vitality are never two mutually exclusive options on some lifestyle multiple choice question. *Both* improve as Christians fast; they are inherently complimentary in a life fully devoted to Christ's lordship.[4]

For those who *actually believe* that Jesus meant what he said, fasting is not an option. He gave specific instructions about fasting

2. "Great Lent."

3. The comprehensive benefits of fasting are well documented in the health literature. See, for example, Persynaki et al., "Unraveling the Metabolic Health Benefits of Fasting Related to Religious Beliefs: A Narrative Review," 14–20.

4. See appendix B for a summary of my food-related testimony.

in the Sermon on the Mount: note that Matthew 6:16 states *"and when you fast"* (not *if* you fast). Jesus also foretold that, after his ascension, his disciples would fast! Three of the four Gospels record this comfort-challenging prophecy and implied command: Matthew 9:15, Mark 2:20, and Luke 5:35. Those texts contain no hint of an opt-out clause because of sugar-withdrawal headaches or caffeine-withdrawal shakes. Christ's disciples are characterized by fasting, especially when major decisions must be made (see Acts 13:2–3 and 14:23).

When I first began to fast monthly, I did not do so to devote myself to prayer. Rather, to my great surprise, prayer flowed almost effortlessly from my soul—as naturally as embarrassing odors flowed from my mouth and other parts of my body.[5] As noted above, I fast primarily because Jesus said his disciples—the *real* ones, *all* of them—would do this! He was, in effect, commanding me (and you) to engage regularly in some form of food abstinence. And I fast because it is profoundly, holistically good for me. Most of all, I fast to hear his voice, to know his heart, and to be surprised by both—again!

HOW LONG SHOULD WE FAST?

Even if we accept fasting as part of the normal Christian life, key questions immediately surface. How much is enough? Does one meal count? What about two meals? Do we all need to fast for forty days to be like Jesus? Is fasting physically dangerous (especially if diabetic, etc.)?[6] So many questions arise about a spiritual discipline Christians in the West know so little about.

---

5. Medical evidence for detoxification of the body through fasting is quite limited, despite detoxing's popularity in the naturopathic world. The following two research summaries are helpful:
- Klein and Kiat, "Detox Diets for Toxin Elimination."
- Genius, "Elimination of Persistent Toxicants."

6. Everyone intending to pursue a lengthy water-only fast should first consult with a medical provider.

Varied answers abound for the how-long question. As noted above, liturgical churches usually fast forty days during the pre-Easter Lenten season. Those who advocate the "Daniel fast" often set a ten-day to twenty-one-day fasting period. Others promote no-food fasts for a limited number of meals. Few, if any, recommend the *no-nothing* fast modelled by Saul of Tarsus (the apostle Paul) when "blinded by the Light" and totally dumbfounded in Damascus (Acts 9:9). Bible-based models are obviously quite diverse,[7] as are medical-based models.[8]

Prior to my 2011-to-2013 weight loss, the longest I ever fasted was one painfully abandoned meal. Early in 2012, however, I became consumed by a novel goal: "I will *tithe* my days through fasting three days this month . . . *every* month!" These were—and remain for me—no-food[9] days of exploring God and my own body, of confronting my cravings and food-focused destructive habits, of marveling at the fact that I rarely feel hungry, especially on day three.

I began embracing (in ignorance[10]) an approach to fasting with some scientific support in both the popular and scientific literature.[11] Apparently three-day fasts with zero or near-zero caloric intake are really good for us! What immediately amazed (and still amazes) me was the clear, centered, and *cravings-free* peace of day three. To date, I have not gone beyond a three-day fast. My spiritual, mental, and physical goals are satisfied, month by month, within those 72-hours. I *always* break my fasts loving Jesus more, feeling food's power over me shattered, and my prayers, thoughts, and goals dominated by God's presence.

7. "Types of Fasting."

8. Seliger, "Is Fasting Healthy?"

9. I typically consume only water and juice.

10. This is a fairly common state of affairs for me when it comes to truly understanding my body.

11. See, for example, the following three sources:
- "The Many Benefits of Fasting."
- Hewitt, "10 Benefits of Fasting that Will Surprise You."
- Salzberg, "Can a 3-day Fast Reset Your Immune System?"

CAN WE TRULY MASTER HUNGER AND CRAVINGS?

People who know my fasting lifestyle have asked how hungry I feel during those three days each month. My honest answer remains, "I'm almost never hungry!" Since I normally eat only two meals[12] a day, I am already "fasting" part of every day. The transition from my normal 16-hour "intermittent" fast[13] to a 72-hour (three-day) fast is largely a hunger-free experience.[14] Honestly, I wrestle more with hunger during non-fasting days than during those special hours of purposeful restraint. Even so, I am very grateful for that breaking-my-fast meal at the end of the three days.

Cravings are not hunger! True hunger is physiological; cravings are usually psychological. God designed food to satisfy our bodies, *not* our minds! Far too many Christians bypass the Great Physician, preferring to self-medicate[15] their inner wounds with food. We *must* understand the purpose of food, for that understanding will empower us to value fasting as God's way to bring holistic healing and comprehensive lifestyle change.

The purpose of *food* is
to push back true hunger,
so I can live and love,
and work and serve,
without weakness or distraction.

The purpose of *fasting* is
to embrace true hunger,
so I can cleanse body and soul,
and fellowship with him who said,
"Man shall not live by bread alone."

---

12. See the section entitled "Tapping the Power of Habit Strength" in chapter 6.

13. For a useful introduction to intermittent fasting, see "Intermittent Fasting (Time-Restricted Eating)."

14. Remember that it was *after* forty days of fasting that hunger strongly impacted Jesus (Matt 4:2).

15. See chapter 13.

Until early 2012, I had little experience with true hunger. Even now, I struggle to distinguish hunger from the powerful pull of habits and the seductive sensation of cravings. I need three full days of fasting to relearn the difference. Those three-day fasts crush my cravings and break my food-focused destructive habits—at least for another month! Giving thanks to God for his provision at the end of day three is an incredible joy.

A FINAL APPEAL

Those who earnestly seek to follow Jesus must incorporate *some* form of food-focused fasting into their lives: view it as part of an authentic Christian life. From a biblical perspective, refusing to follow Christ into the emptiness of fasting is as unthinkable as refusing to follow him into the death-waters of baptism. Today, *"when the bridegroom"* is gone (Luke 5:35), our Lord is calling his followers to live out a fasting lifestyle.

11

Fasting and Suffering
Knowing Him the Other Way

"God had one son on earth without sin, but never one without suffering." Saint Augustine[1]

KNOWING HIM FULLY

IN PHILIPPIANS 3:10, PAUL revealed his deepest motivation: *"That I may know him, and the power of his resurrection, and the fellowship of his sufferings, being made conformable unto his death"* (KJV). This is likely one of the most *partially* quoted verses in the New Testament, the words trailing off rapidly after the word *resurrection*. Many Christians sincerely seek to know Jesus—but on their terms, not his. They long to feel *"the power of his resurrection,"* attracted by the "tingles" and "do-dads" and "Holy Ghost power" displays. Without question, the power of Christ's resurrection must have been awesome! Sealed stone rolling one way, soldiers sprawled like dead men the other way, grave-opening earthquake, and blinding

1. https://www.brainyquote.com/quotes/saint_augustine_148526.

light everywhere! Yes! I want to know that Jesus . . . in *that* power![2] Sign me up; I want to know this resurrected all-powerful Christ!

Sadly, most Philippians 3:10 sermons proclaimed from western pulpits fail to declare the full passion of this verse. Few preachers know what to do with *"the fellowship of his sufferings."* Bluntly stated, most Christians fear, dread, and rebuke suffering. How can we suffer *and* walk in victory? Are we to actually embrace suffering? For many, suffering signals that something has gone horribly wrong in their Christian walk. No one publishes books explaining the *7 Keys to Successful Suffering.* Christian publishers typically seek manuscripts that appeal to the power-hungry, not the suffering-hungry! What, then, shall we do with part C of Philippians 3:10?

Knowing only *"the power of his resurrection"* is comparable to knowing only one side of a brilliant, priceless coin—the kind of stunning coin that would drive a man to sell all he owns to possess it (similar to Matt 13:46). Imagine a neurotic coin collector—let's call him Fred—who feared to examine the "tails" of his treasured collection. Fred would never know the true value of his heads-only collection, no matter how often he studied it. Even the face value of many coins is stated only on its back side!

A TROUBLING STATEMENT

The most troubling statement in all of Scripture, at least for me, is found in Matthew chapter 7. Describing the final judgment, Jesus warned that many will try to enter the kingdom of heaven, but he will tell them to go away. They will object (Matt 7:22), citing their use of spiritual power in his name as evidence they merited special favor: *"Lord, Lord, did we not prophesy in your name, and cast out demons in your name, and do many mighty works in your name?"* His stunning reply will be *"I never knew you"* (Matt 7:23). How is that possible? *Jesus knows everything . . . and everyone!* These

2. Note that the multitude in John 6:26 followed Jesus to get some more of his miracle bread.

miracle workers will be rejected by the greatest Miracle Worker of all time—astounding!

The warning is clear, compelling, and frankly terrifying. Like poor Fred the neurotic coin collector, some Christians strive to know only the "heads" of Christ's resurrection power, never fully embracing the "tails" of suffering for him and with him. Unfortunately, the Lord will likely declare on that day that he never knew them. The only way to avoid this horror is to invest the time (and bear the pain) needed to know him *fully* through sharing in his sufferings.

SUFFERING IS BIBLICAL

The *gospel* of Jesus Christ is, by definition, *good news*. But that news is costly! It cost Jesus his life. And it continues to cost his followers; some suffer great loss and pain in order to know him fully. The not-so-fine print in this good-news offer is loaded with references to suffering. The following verses sample the "terms-and-conditions-apply" clauses in the good news message:

- Colossians 1:24: *"Now I rejoice in my sufferings for your sake, and in my flesh I am filling up what is lacking in Christ's afflictions for the sake of his body, that is, the church."*

- 2 Timothy 2:10–12: *"Therefore I endure everything for the sake of the elect, that they also may obtain the salvation that is in Christ Jesus with eternal glory. The saying is trustworthy . . . if we endure,*[3] *we will also reign with him."*

- 1 Peter 1:6–7: *"In this* [salvation] *you rejoice, though now for a little while, if necessary, you have been grieved by various trials, so that the tested genuineness of your faith—more precious than gold that perishes though it is tested by fire—may be found to result in praise and glory and honor at the revelation of Jesus Christ."*

---

3. This term is translated *suffer* in the KJV.

Suffering for the faith[4] is deeply engrained in the New Testament message, though we might wish it otherwise. It is one of God's spiritual-discipline "tools;" he uses suffering to perfect Christ's image deep inside of us. The experience of suffering forces us to focus on eternity and on Christ Jesus our Lord! Paul powerfully argued that we endure suffering so we will *"not lose heart. . . . For this light momentary affliction is preparing for us an eternal weight of glory beyond all comparison, as we look not to the things that are seen but to the things that are unseen"* (2 Cor 4:16–18). As people of faith, we focus (by faith) on things that cannot be verified by senses or sciences. In our present struggles, sufferings, and pain, we must remain focused on the invisible, the eternal.

FASTING AS SELF-IMPOSED SUFFERING

This chapter's title promises a link between fasting and suffering. The link, in my view, boldly confronts the unbiblical conclusion that suffering is evil, not beneficial—something dark and ugly, not beautiful and life-giving. Most western Christians have little experience with persecution and suffering, and are happy to keep it that way. But they dare not neglect those challenging verses (above) that describe suffering as part of the normal Christian life. Suffering paves the "narrow way" (see Matt 7:13–14, KJV) that leads to spiritual victory and intimacy with Christ.

Trust me, I have no masochistic desire to suffer. I do not hit my head on walls (at least not intentionally), and I never tie a "Please Kick Me" sign on my back belt loop. But I have discovered, painfully, that I draw closer to my Savior when fasting than when waddling out of an all-you-can-possibly-consume eatery, burdened with stupid calories and gluttony's guilt.

Day to day, I never really suffer for Jesus—not like those in the persecuted church around the world. No one verbally abuses me because I bow to pray over a restaurant meal. And I have never been arrested for entering a church building. To be transparent,

4. 1 Pet 2:19–21 clearly differentiates suffering for the sake of righteousness and suffering as a result of stupidity.

I am happy I am not actively suffering for my faith! But then, his Word pulls me back to biblical reality. What about knowing Jesus in the hard times? What about walking with him in pain and shame? I *really* do want to reign with him forever! I *really* do want to hear him say, *"Well done!"* (Matt 25:21, 23). How can I qualify for that summary judgment without suffering?

Fasting offers Christians in the West a brief exposure to knowing Christ the *other* way. And for that reason, I treasure my three-day fasts each month. The miracle-working power of his resurrection is certainly attractive, no doubt. But I passionately want to know him—and be known by him—the *other* way, too!

Do I really suffer while fasting? Honestly, not much! Yes, sleeping becomes a greater challenge. Yes, physical weakness increases throughout those days. Yes, I feel the cold more during my wintertime fasts. These mild discomforts are as close to suffering for him as I get, at least for now in the United States. Harder days are coming. Persecution may soon ravage our communities. Until then, I will continue to embrace fasting in my desire to know him the other way—in the *"fellowship of his sufferings."*

12

Fasting and Weight Loss
Avoiding Self-Deception

"Lying to ourselves is more deeply ingrained than lying to others." Fyodor Dostoevsky[1]

CONFESSIONS OF A FAST-ER ENDING A FAST

I CHOSE TO START this chapter while ending one of my three-day fasts. As I write this paragraph, I feel awesome, centered, peaceful. An added bonus, I saw a digital display on my scales this morning I have not seen for almost two years. I had gained a few pounds since my all-time adult low in March 2013. Those last few unwanted pounds—stubborn offspring of Indulgence and Weakness—just refused to leave home! This fast, supported by weeks of restraint, apparently delivered the needed eviction notice to those naughty children. Yes, fasting just *might* be the magic bullet of weight loss! Just stop eating for three full days and the scales start singing beautifully . . . again! Yet I have learned to not trust its seductive song.

1. https://www.goodreads.com/quotes/317999-lying-to-ourselves-is-more-deeply-ingrained-than-lying-to.

Tonight I broke my three-day fast with a salad. Profoundly grateful for the mixed greens (calories) in my bowl, I tentatively re-entered the world of normal eating. Only it was not completely normal: I chose to leave about a third of the salad for tomorrow evening's meal. I ate to supply calories for my mildly depleted biosystem. I did not prepare that salad in response to my inner cravings, just as I did not begin this fast to lose weight.

DECEPTION-FRIENDLY BELIEFS

Weight loss would be an admirable goal for almost 70 percent of Americans[2] who fall into the overweight (or higher[3]) category. You may be among them. Is fasting the solution to your weight problem? This chapter briefly examines five statements that, at first glance, seem appealing. Their collective appeal is, however, an invitation to self-deception about weight loss. My greatest weight-loss struggle has *always* been mental, not physical. My greatest temptation has *always* been self-deceptive—and ultimately, self-destructive—thoughts and attitudes about food and me.

Not biologically trained, I do not claim to understand the biomedical mechanics of fasting.[4] Details about metabolism rates and the body's switch from burning glucose to burning fat continue to elude me. Consequently, this chapter focuses on *attitudes* toward food, weight loss, and fasting: these I *do* understand! Our belief systems, what we *hold* to be true, strongly influence our behaviors. Unfortunately, the greater the gap between what we *believe* to be true and the truth, the more we are embracing some form of self-deception.

---

2. See "Overweight & Obesity Statistics."

3. At 5 feet 9 inches tall, I would be classified as *obese* if I weighed between 203 and 270 pounds: above 270 pounds, I would fall in *class 3: morbidly obese*. For additional details, see "Defining Adult Overweight and Obesity."

4. I urge a just-to-be-safe consultation with a medical provider before fasting. Excellent resources on fasting are listed at the end of this chapter.

MYTH 1: GOD DESIGNED FASTING FOR WEIGHT LOSS

The biblical theology of weight loss makes for really quick reading! Scripture has almost nothing to say about losing weight. The Bible does contain a few references to fat people (Ps 73:7; Jer 5:28; Jas 5:5); the obese people identified in these particular passages are described negatively. Still, trying to locate any command, including the command to fast, for the sake of weight loss is futile. Both Old Testament commands to fast and New Testament examples of fasting have everything to do with the condition of the heart, not the girth of the waist.

MYTH 2: YOUR LOWEST FASTING WEIGHT IS YOUR NEW NORMAL WEIGHT

Seasoned fast-ers know they lose fluids more rapidly than they lose fat (or muscle), especially during the first day or two of an extended fast.[5] The scales begin to record deceptively appealing numbers, even though the fast-ers are downing more water than usual. This fact allows those hawking the latest diet fads to boast about dramatic "weight" losses during the first seven to ten days. The diuretics[6] in dieting "supplements" work as intended, creating the illusion of miraculous *fat*-reducing success!

During a three-day fast, I typically drop five to six pounds, invoking fantasies of a fat-killing magic bullet. Yet I know that fasting (like dieting) is an abnormal state. My lowest fasting weight is *never* sustainable for the rest of that month. Even when eating with moderation, I will weigh more a week *after* ending a fast than just *before* I break it. My low-point weight at the end of a fast, though tempting, demands a serious reality check!

5. Corleone, "How Much Weight Will I Lose on a Water Fast?"
6. See, for example, "What's in Your Diet Pills?"

MYTH 3: FASTING IS BIBLICAL, THEREFORE IT IS SAFE

Fasting is, indeed, biblical, but Old Testament fasts were typically brief ones. The Day of Atonement (*Yom Kippur*: see Lev 23:26–32) was the only fast required by the Old Testament law.[7] Even when special fasts were called (for example, Esth 4:16), none were long-term events. Similarly, the fasts described in the New Testament were not extensive: none were the forty-day variety that prepared Christ for his public ministry. While he remains our ultimate role model, Jesus never required his disciples to emulate his severe fast.

Weeks-long, water-only fasts create potential health risks that must be taken seriously. Internal organs can be seriously impacted by prolonged fasts. Fast-ers who are not particularly healthy at the start of such an endeavor should seek prior medical advice and secure real-time supervision. Even healthy fast-ers should build up to extensive fasting periods, much like people develop fitness over weeks of physical training.[8]

MYTH 4: FASTING IS EASY BECAUSE IT REQUIRES NO EFFORT

Like aging, fasting requires no effort whatsoever: do nothing and simply watch the time pass. *Simple* is not, however, *easy*—especially when making a commitment that melds together spirit and body. Fasting is *never* easy: the fast-er must accommodate the reality of declining energy levels and periods of schedule-impacting weakness. Even those otherwise good-for-you physical workouts—both strength-training and cardio-training sessions—should be seriously moderated while fasting. I honor my fasts through significantly lighter workouts.

The most challenging aspect of fasting occurs when I unexpectedly encounter the social pressure to eat with others.[9] Do I

7. "Fasting and Fast-Days."

8. It is possible, perhaps even likely, that Jesus fasted often during his silent years, prior to his baptism by John and the Spirit's anointing.

9. I plan each monthly fast to avoid scheduled dining events. When that is not possible, I either shorten my fast accordingly or try to move the meeting

break my fast to join this group at a restaurant, or that individual wanting time with me at lunch? Social events become hard decision points; each must be judged individually. I am reluctant to tell anyone other than my wife when I am fasting; honestly, I struggle to know what to do in such situations.[10] Still, I have learned that *social expectations do not define authentic living!*

MYTH (SORT OF) 5: FASTING BREAKS THE POWER OF FOOD

Unlike the previous four myths, this statement is part myth, part truth. One of my discoveries since 2012 is fasting's amazing impact on food's powerful grip. Fasting does indeed break the power of food in my life—*for a while*. Viscerally and spiritually, I sense the power of food shattering. Afterward, I eat because I need the calories, deeply grateful to God for them. I do *not* eat because I crave food, at least not for a few weeks!

Unfortunately, cravings slowly return as food gradually, persistently re-exerts its pull. How I wish a single fast could permanently break the power of food. This, however, has not been my experience. I must repeatedly empty myself to break its power—again! I view this as a visceral metaphor of my need to return repeatedly to my Savior in repentance for succumbing (again!) to the power of sin. *"But thanks be to God, who gives us the victory through our Lord Jesus Christ"* (1 Cor 15:57). Victory through the painful process of fasting is a treasured gift!

---

away from a normal meal time so I can drink black coffee.

10. Ironically, fasting can generate spiritual pride when the fast-er focuses more on the process than the Lord of the process. Those who fast extensively must guard their hearts, lest they become puffed up with their "success" in this ultimate emptying experience.

THREE USEFUL WEB SITES

- *Diet Myth or Truth: Fasting Is Effective for Weight Loss:* http://www.webmd.com/diet/features/diet-myth-truth-fasting-effective-weight-loss#1

- *Effect of Alternate-Day Fasting on Weight Loss, Weight Maintenance, and Cardioprotection among Metabolically Healthy Obese Adults: A Randomized Clinical Trial:* http://jamanetwork.com/journals/jamainternalmedicine/article-abstract/2623528

- *Fasting Tips for Weight Loss:* http://www.livestrong.com/article/148906-fasting-tips-for-weight-loss/

13

Obesity and Self-Medication
Surrendering Self-Hatred

"If you had a person in your life treating you the way you treat yourself, you would have gotten rid of them a long time ago." Cheri Huber[1]

BACKGROUND

I CONSIDERED OMITTING THIS chapter after finishing the first three units. The chapter's focus seemed out of place in this "Sometimes Hungry" unit. The title does not include the word *fasting*, while the sub-title contains a strongly provocative term: *self-hatred*. After considerable internal debate and prayer, I concluded the chapter is essential—at least for some readers. If you are not one of those readers[2]—if you are not struggling with obesity and its associated destructive emotions, feel free to skip forward to chapter 14!

---

1. https://www.goodreads.com/quotes/293404-if-you-had-a-person-in-your-life-treating-you.

2. And no one you love is, either.

SELF-HATRED . . . REALLY?

Perhaps the term *self-hatred* is overstated. After all, Christians are supposed to be loving people and are profoundly loved by God. And he remains constantly committed to their eternal salvation. Still, the sixty-billion-dollar[3] diet industry thrives on an endless supply of deeply dissatisfied (*desperate?*) people—Christians included! All serious dieters intensely dislike (*hate?*) their bodies (*themselves*) so much they are willing to invest their hard-earned money to buy the latest, beautifully advertised "miracle." Why do they so willingly throw their money to the wind? I am convinced (as suggested by the parenthetical terms above) they hate themselves and are desperately looking for a way out of their misery.

Obesity is at epidemic levels among Christians; both a visual survey of most congregations on any given Sunday and recently published research support this conclusion.[4] Those who attend church regularly are *at least* as obese (perhaps far more so) as the general population, which is now almost 40-percent obese.[5] Churches are filled with (and led by) a troubling percentage of spiritually transformed people characterized, unfortunately, by no food restraint.[6] And in *almost all* of those churches, the sin of gluttony—yes, *sin*—is never mentioned; Body Mass Index[7] (BMI) is *never* addressed as a spiritual concern. Compounding the problem, Christians typically celebrate major church events through excessive food intake,[8] underscoring the moral vacuum created by pastoral silence! Sadly, many of those Christian leaders who loudly condemn drug and alcohol abuse never mention food addiction.

---

3. See "What the $60 Billion Weight Loss Industry Doesn't Want You to Know." For another perspective, see "100 Million Dieters, $20 Billion: The Weight-Loss Industry by the Numbers."

4. See the editorial-type summary: "Fat in Church."

5. Healy, "Nearly 4 in 10 US Adults Are Now Obese, CDC Says."

6. They may exercise admirable restraint in *other* areas of their lives.

7. The body's percentage of fat, compared to its total weight: See "BMI (Body Mass Index): What Is BMI?"

8. Cline and Ferraro, "Does Religion Increase the Prevalence and Incidence of Obesity in Adulthood?" 269–81.

At one point in the past, I saw a woman at church who could barely walk; she was carrying the equivalent of another person with every step. My heart ached for her—and for her family! If opening her heart to a trusted, confidence-holding friend, she would (I believe) admit how frustrated and defeated she feels, and how physically and emotionally exhausted she remains most of the time. Her pain (*I know!*) torments all the more intensely in a spiritual environment that promises abundant life, promotes moral discipline, and proclaims holistic healing.

A central premise of this difficult-to-write chapter is that morbidly obese people hate themselves. At some deeply buried, heavily bunkered, rarely entered level, they are trapped by their self-hatred. Yet most hate admitting it even more. This was my own experience for decades—partially *wasted* decades—of my life, starting in third grade.[9] Jolly fat people do not really exist! This stereotype is perpetuated by some (certainly not all) obese people who have learned how to mask their inner pain with outer humor. While inner pain is certainly not the unique experience of the obese, they attempt to insulate themselves—literally—from their pain!

TWO STREAMS—ONE SAD SELF-MEDICATED OUTCOME

Obesity is the all-too visible byproduct of an inner dysfunction originating (in my view) from two closely related "streams" of experience. Those "swimming" (floating?) in Stream A have discovered that an earlier traumatic experience or emotional wound[10] hurts less when they are eating. In essence, they *self-medicate* through food intake to numb their persistent pain. Sadly, they resemble their hurting neighbors who self-medicate with starva-

---

9. See the section entitled "Resolutions: New Year vs. Old Year" in chapter 6.

10. Perhaps a childhood or adolescent event that now defines them. Many sexually abused children unconsciously attempt to defend themselves from further attack by defensive eating, striving to make themselves less attractive to the predators in their lives. See, for example, Khazan, "The Second Assault."

tion-type eating disorders, drugs, alcohol, and sex: all seeking the same temporary relief from pain. Ultimately, *every* expression of self-medication only intensifies the pain—visibly so for the food addict.

Those "swimming" in the Stream B may be largely free of past trauma; they simply have been seduced by eating's stimulation of their brains' pleasure center.[11] They have become addicted to that feels-so-good sensation, and can't wait to experience that mildly euphoric state again.[12] Non-obese people, in general, *eat to live* and respond appropriately to the brain's "you've-had-enough" satiety signals. Others, unfortunately, *live to eat,* eagerly embracing a food-focused, addictive lifestyle. And the fatter they grow, year by year, the more they turn to food for temporary relief from their growing sense of pain and self-loathing. The irony in this circular, self-defeating pattern of behavior is stunning!

FOOD AND THE VICIOUS CYCLE

This chapter argues that obese people regularly seek pain relief in the wrong place. The "pharmacy" (including the fridge) of self-medicated relief from soul-level pain is *always* the wrong place! Only a brutally honest, transparent encounter with the healing "Balm of Gilead" can heal pain that deep. Food is intended for the gut, not for "the sin-sick soul."[13]

A vicious cycle of self-hatred entraps the food-addicted self-medicators. They may briefly escape their inner pain by consuming hundreds of unneeded calories, inflating BMI figures, and intensifying despair when they do glance at themselves in the mirror. As noted earlier, the brain releases opiate-like endorphins throughout their far-too-long meals. These can overwhelm the brain's normal "no-thanks-I'm-full" signal.[14] And the vicious cycle continues.

11. "Food Opiates: Are You Addicted?"

12. "Food Addiction."

13. See the lyrics to this public-domain hymn at https://hymnary.org/text/sometimes_i_feel_discouraged_spiritual.

14. Kenny, "Is Obesity an Addiction?"

SURRENDERING SELF-HATRED

Recovery from obesity requires healing from, and finding deep satisfaction in, a Source other than food. Dieting *never* heals self-hatred; failure inevitably follows all that misdirected effort and expense. Pounds are ultimately added and self-hatred is intensified when the bathroom scale is finally allowed to tell its unwanted tale. While self-hatred yields deep despair, inner healing yields life-transformation and hope!

My sincere plea for those trapped in morbid obesity is to surrender *all* self-judgment, including self-hatred and its related despair, to Christ's Lordship. Total surrender is, after all, the essence of baptism: dead to my failed lordship, alive to his reign in my life. When truly living under his Lordship, I am just a *doulos*—a simple "*servant,*" to use Paul's term (for example, in Rom 1:1; Phil 1:1). Living under his Lordship, *I have no right to feel something about myself that he does not feel for me.*

Romans 14:4(a) asks, "*Who are you to pass judgment on the servant of another? It is before his own master that he stands or falls.*" I do not have the right to judge (as in hate) myself if I am truly dead, truly no longer my own master. Christianity's lofty goal of "dying to self" must begin with a simple renunciation of my own self-mastery . . . of my own lordship. A Christian *must* surrender self-mastery to Christ, for only he "*is able to make him stand*" (Rom 14:4(c)).

My advice to obese Christians? Actively renounce all fraudulent lordship in the context of food. For thirty days, at *every meal,* begin by offering an empty plate to your Lord, asking him to fill it with what is essential for your health—and to fill your soul with his healing presence. Then serve (not *fill*) that plate at the stove, microwave, or refrigerator—*not* at the table (where far too many extra calories temptingly await within arm's reach). Take every bite under his Lordship! And *never* return to the stove for self-inflicted "seconds." In the context of recovery, gluttony is idolatry and self-hatred is rebellion. Our Lord urges us to action: "*Learn from me . . . and you will find rest for your souls*" (Matt 11:29).

UNIT 5

Painful Joys

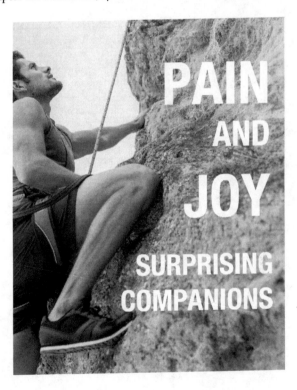

14

"Pain 101"

Enrollment Is Mandatory

"Life is pain, Highness. Anyone who says differently is selling something." William Goldman[1]

PAIN: FROM DAY ONE

THE NEWBORN HAS JUST been rudely squeezed out of her warm, dark, quiet environment: it was "practically perfect in every way" except for its increasingly cramped space. Violently evicted from the only home she has ever known, she's overwhelmed by numbing cold, blinding light, and deafening sounds. And she *hurts all over* on this most awful day 1 of the rest of her life. Welcome to Pain 101, little lady! You are now officially enrolled, and will remain so for life!

1. https://www.goodreads.com/quotes/1387-life-is-pain-highness-anyone-who-says-differently-is-selling.

Owies, boo-boos, and similar terms of supposed comfort provide an intriguing backdrop for this topic of pain. Parents and adult care-givers use such terms to simultaneously label pain and sympathize with the hurting (*screaming!*) child. Each of the amazingly complex childhood developmental skills—like scooting, crawling, standing, walking, and dancing—are initially accompanied by more painful failures than joyful successes. The persistence children display daily in the face of inevitable pain belies behaviorism's flawed learning theory that argues we repeat behaviors for which we are rewarded, and avoid those that generate painful outcomes.[2] Unless they are deeply wounded internally—in their spirits, by parental abuse, those falling, screaming children will (eventually) stop crying, get up, and *try it again!*

PAIN: THE EVER-PRESENT TEACHER

Many view pain as some enemy from which escape is the only reasonable goal; some orient their entire lives toward escapism. Ironically, their persistent desire to escape pain entraps them in a risk-free life or a slow, drug-imprisoned death. Pain, like hunger, is not an enemy. It can be, however, an amazingly effective teacher! Some of life's greatest lessons demand pain's careful, persistent instruction. Touched a hot stove top? *Lesson: ALWAYS check the stovetop's temperature before touching it!* Forgot to apply sunscreen before that magical day at the beach? *Lesson: ALWAYS remember the sun screen!*

Pain's memorable lessons shape our future behavior far longer than any classroom instruction. Pain *also* serves as a reliable internal warning device. The book[3] *Pain: The Gift Nobody Wants* contains an intriguing statement on the cover: "WARNING: *Life without pain could really hurt you!*" We have nerve endings throughout our bodies for a reason: our protection! Lepers lose fingers, toes, and other extremities because they can no longer feel

2. See, for example, Nayak, "Behaviorism as a Theory of Personality: A Critical Look."

3. Brand and Yancey, *Pain: The Gift Nobody Wants.*

pain in them. Pain is God's gift to us, signaling that something is wrong; a threat to our wellbeing is imminent. As I explain in chapter 15, God used pain I could no longer ignore in one part of my body to expose the cancer threatening my life in another location that was still pain free. Ignorance, not pain, is one of life's greatest enemies.

PAIN: THE CONSTANT IN PHYSICAL TRAINING

Mentally healthy people do not enjoy pain; they do not seek it out just because they feel so good when the pain stops. Still, pain is present in all physical disciplines (cardio and strength training, even fasting). Recall that the chapters in units 2 and 3 focused on cardio and strength training. Pain is the common factor in the physical training described in those chapters. In fact, we cannot improve performance without pain. Serious athletes welcome pain and the truth in Robert Allen's profound statement: "Everything you want is just outside your comfort zone."[4] World records in athletic events are *never* set by comfortable, pain-free people!

In *cardio* training, pain is the inevitable by-product of increased endurance (how *long*) and accelerated speed[5] (how *fast*). Ideally, the discomfort (that is, the pain!) during the pursuit of greater levels of fitness is moderate in intensity. No falls! No twisted ankles or knees! No risky maneuvers on cardio equipment! A training accident can set you back weeks to months in pursuit of your fitness goals. Steady pushing without heroics will generate motivating results over several months. Even so, none of the thousands of steps required during that process will ever be completely pain free: this truth constitutes another DWI.[6]

During *strength* training, pain is also a dominant, recurring experience. This experience centers on weight (how *heavy*) and

4. Hansen and Allen. *The One Minute Millionaire: The Enlightened Way to Wealth.*

5. This includes increased difficulty through resistance and incline settings on various cardio equipment.

6. (Deal With It) See chapter 8.

reps (how *many* . . . before temporary exhaustion). By definition, the process of breaking muscles down is painful; yes, they *must* break down (somewhat) before they can rebuild stronger than before. My first utterance after finishing a set on many lifts is "Oouuw!" The pain is real but short-lived. Still, the pervasive soreness I feel two days later (especially if I have not been consistently lifting hard) comes *really* close to pain!

Discerning the various types of exercise-generated pain is essential for those in training. While our natural tendency is to avoid pain, those who take training seriously take pain in stride—literally. They have become well acquainted with it and, to some extent, *depend* on it. Distance runners know that pain will join them at some point during their runs—sooner rather than later for the less fit. And weight-lifters know *very* well "the burn" in their targeted muscles after several reps with heavy weight. The challenge is to continue to keep pain in its place (under personal authority), day after day, while never ignoring it completely. Pain must be shown *some* respect, especially if it is screaming from a torn muscle or a strained knee joint.

I occasionally feel discomfort/pain in the lateral (outer) side of my right knee, especially after two sets of calf raises[7] with heavy weight. Typically, this is a transient joint pain, lasting only a few minutes; I usually push on—but doing upper body lifts for a while—and quickly find that my knee is pain free again. Pain on the medial (inside) of my right knee is another matter! Occasionally joining me on the treadmill or walking track, *that* pain can radically curtail my workouts for some time. I have learned the hard way that if my medial-side knee pain does not stop in three to four minutes, I stop![8]

In my experience, *experience* is the only reliable guide for determining if training pain should be respected as a serious warning, or treated as an irritant that I must push through. I take joint pain seriously, muscle pain less so. Yet I know that muscles and

---

7. See "Standing Calf Raises."

8. Fortunately, this knee pain has not hampered my cardio training for almost three years, as of this writing.

cartilage can tear, and ligaments can become inflamed—especially as I age. Even servants are heard by rulers if they speak consistently and urgently. Woe be to the ruler, however, who allows his or her servants to command (see Prov 19:10).

LESSONS TAUGHT IN PAIN 101

My most important lesson learned while enrolled in Pain 101 is that enrollment is mandatory and continuous; this course offers no withdrawal period and only one (final) exam. In this context, Sidney Harris[9] sarcastically observed, "Never take life seriously. Nobody gets out alive anyway."

More specifically, Pain 101 has taught me to continuously employ moderation, sound judgement, and limited risk-taking in many pursuits—especially in my fitness training and fasting. If I suddenly max out my exercise efforts after days-to-weeks of layoff, pain will dominate my life for days. Two "S"s—Slow and Steady— allow me to achieve long-term fitness goals while keeping pain in the teacher's quarters.

Pain is not the enemy! Pain-free living as a life goal is the enemy. Sitting on the couch, eating junk food, and doing nothing are certainly pain-free activities. But type 2 diabetes or heart disease will eventually move in as an unwelcomed family member. Embracing the reality of pain on *my* terms (in the gym or on the road/ track) is the only effective strategy for passing this non-elective course.

---

9. https://www.goodreads.com/quotes/384921-never-take-life-seriously-nobody-gets-out-alive-anyway.

15

Pain and Joy
Paradoxically Compatible

"Blessed are you when others revile you and persecute you and utter all kinds of evil against you falsely on my account. Rejoice and be glad." Jesus Christ (Matt 5:11)

A "PAINFUL" BACKDROP

I DELIVERED MY MOST challenging-to-preach sermon in early October 2014. The event was our retirement farewell chapel service at the Bible school in South Africa where my wife, Rosie, and I served for thirteen years. Dear friends from the school (students, faculty, and staff) and area churches gathered to honor our investment in their classrooms, offices, pulpits, and lives. Their comments continue to buffer against unbidden memories of situations I should have handled better, initiatives for God I could have pursued, prayers I should have prayed, etc., etc.

My most treasured memory of that day was the grace of God I experienced while speaking. Less than an hour before standing to preach, I was sitting in my doctor's office receiving the big "C" (for *Cancer*) verdict, based on his recent medical tests. The providential intervention that led to my first meeting with Dr. Naude the previous week culminated with his informed hunch that I had bladder cancer. Exploratory surgery was essential: "How about tomorrow?" he asked. "Sure," I replied, then drove to preach my farewell message!

During that sermon, "Keeping the main thing the main thing," I challenged those present to affirm that preaching repentance and forgiveness of sins (Luke 24:47) *must* remain the dominant message of the Church.[1] Throughout that exhortation from my heart, I was keenly aware that the Holy Spirit was carrying me . . . calmly . . . through what should have been an emotionally overwhelming morning. While challenging my students with this ultimate lesson in biblical priorities, I was only days away from discovering one of the most important lessons of my own life.

ONE LIFE-TRANSFORMING LESSON . . . IN TWO PARTS

Pain drove me to my family doctor one morning in September, 2014; that unscheduled visit set in motion the process reviewed above. Pain also featured prominently in the two emergency surgeries that followed the initial surgery to remove two cancerous tumors. And, though somewhat controlled pharmaceutically, pain accompanied me home for the weeks of healing that followed. That healing process was complicated by uncertainty and confusion about my future medical treatment. Such are, I believe, the shared experiences of almost all cancer patients.

What caught me totally by surprise was the impact this experience had on me spiritually. Hurting, confused, and scared, I became small again—helpless and *painfully* aware that I needed my Father. The first half of this two-part lesson became crystal clear: *Pain draws the trusting believer close to the Father's heart.* God had not let me down or disappointed me—even when I suspected (just

---

1. I still believe this! And *anything* that threatens to reduce our effectiveness in proclaiming that message must be confronted, repented of, and rejected. This *certainly* includes the undisciplined sins of sloth and gluttony.

before my third surgery in twenty-four hours) that I might die in hospital. My Father had intervened . . . using pain . . . to save my life! The more I reflected on his providential care during those early post-hospital days, the more my heart was "tenderized" by his awesome presence.

Father had my best in view throughout this process! I was pulled, by pain, closer to him than I had been in years. Some friends perceived Satan's cruel hand at work in this crisis. Their perspective offered no comfort, however; in fact, it conflicted sharply with the internal spiritual remodeling God was doing in me. In the weeks following my five-day hospital adventure, I was too much in love with Jesus to care what deceitful scheme my enemy had planned for me. Whatever it may have been, it didn't work!

For sure, the first half of my great lesson surprised me: I was persistently pulled to Father's heart by the lingering impact of pain and threat. The second half of this lesson was a total shock: *joy is the unexpected byproduct of that journey.* Yes, *joy!* It came bubbling up inside of me, like the restless red mass in my mother's old "lava lamp." The closer I got to Jesus, still struggling with fear, confusion, and pain, the more this unexpected joy dominated my recovery. Instead of unending tearful brokenness in his presence, I was flooded with delightful joy knowing I was *"accepted in the beloved"* (Eph 1:6, KJV). That arms-wide-open welcome still overwhelms me, still soaks my mind and soul with fresh waves of joy!

PAINFUL FAITHFUL AFFLICTION

I do not like a few parts of the Bible very much. As I child, I enthusiastically sang that "every promise in the Book is mine." Now I understand that I do not want some of those promises! Hebrews 12:5–11,[2] for example, contains a promise I have never "claimed"

2. *"And have you forgotten the exhortation that addresses you as sons? 'My son, do not regard lightly the discipline of the Lord, nor be weary when reproved by him. For the Lord disciplines the one he loves, and chastises every son whom he receives.' It is for discipline that you have to endure. God is treating you as sons. . . . he disciplines us for our good, that we may share his holiness. For the*

because it promises pain. *Yes,* I desperately long to be God's son—I love that promise, especially as phrased in John 1:12–13.[3] *No,* I do not want to be ignored (disowned) as a spiritually illegitimate child (*"bastard"* in the KJV)! But spiritual discipline is painful; I honestly do not like this "promise" of divine discipline! Even so, I have renewed my trust in the always-fair, always-loving Father of this painful process, so I am learning—again—to welcome his discipline when it comes.

Normally the New Testament illustrates, explains, and illumines the sometimes cryptic passages in the Old Testament. However, several months after my surgery, I encountered a passage in Psalm 119 (verses 65 through 75) that offers profound perspective on God's process of spiritual discipline.[4] This passage (with some verses omitted) states:

> You have dealt well with your servant, O Lord, according to your word. . . . Before I was afflicted I went astray, but now I keep your word. . . . It is good for me that I was afflicted, that I might learn your statutes. . . . I know, O Lord, that your rules are righteous, and that in faithfulness you have afflicted me.

My Father's faithful affliction performed wonders deep within my soul. He did not leave me alone, did not allow me to go *"astray"*—to wander from his heart in my delusional self-sufficiency. The "affliction" of cancer he allowed me to experience deflated my ego and shrunk my arrogance; it exorcized pride and humbled me . . . again. My affliction mercifully drove me back to the narrow way that leads to life,[5] and restored my deep, bubbling joy in being his son.

---

moment all discipline seems painful rather than pleasant, but later it yields the peaceful fruit of righteousness to those who have been trained by it."

3. *"To all who did receive him, who believed in his name, he gave the right to become children of God, who were born, not of blood nor of the will of the flesh nor of the will of man, but of God."*

4. See Heb 12.

5. See Matt 7:14, KJV.

PARADOXICALLY COMPATIBLE

"All discipline seems painful" at the time, *"but later..."* (Heb 12:11).
I can now see with some clarity the truth that had been frustrat-
ingly fuzzy: there is always a *"later"* in God's parental intervention
in our lives. I now confess that he has *"dealt well"* with me. *"It is
good for me that I was afflicted,"* for his intervention in 2014 constantly reminds me that I am truly his son. Though I may child-
ishly, foolishly wish it were not so, my Father is not reluctant to
use my pain for his purposes. And his purposes *always* generate
life-transforming joy!

Pain and joy: these radically distinct experiences are not
incompatible. For the child of God, paradox is the norm—as in
*"whoever would save his life will lose it, but whoever loses his life for
my sake will find it"* (Matt 16:25). Pain and joy are intricately, paradoxically linked for those who know they are deeply loved—for
those who understand they are being disciplined, not punished.[6]

Only death will enable me to see with perfect clarity the full
impact of God's painful intervention in my life. I *know* that my
response to 2014's pain, embarrassment, and confusion have profoundly impacted my life in these few intervening years. And I
suspect that my response to his loving discipline has in some way
brought him glory: a thought that remains staggering, humbling,
and overwhelming!

---

6. This chapter indirectly raises an important question: Should I intervene
in the pain or suffering of another person? Stated differently, if a person is
being afflicted by the Lord (Ps 119), would my intervention thwart God's purposes? Of course, it could not do so! Nothing within my paltry power to bless
another person could possibly offset Father's intervention in his or her life. On
the other hand, my power to bless another may constitute God's beneficent
intervention. Prov 3:27 states, *"Do not withhold good from those to whom it is
due, when it is in your power to do it."* Similarly, Heb 13:16 admonishes, *"Do not
neglect to do good and to share what you have, for such sacrifices are pleasing to
God."* As we have opportunity, we should focus on being a source of blessing to
others, as plainly directed in Scripture (see Gal 6:10), and leave the business of
correction through affliction in God's hands.

16

Sacrificial Joy
Paradox on the Road "Less Traveled By"

"Two roads diverged in a wood
and I—I took the one less traveled by,
and that has made all the difference." Robert Frost[1]

FROM ANIMAL TO HUMAN SACRIFICES

IN LEVITICUS,[2] GOD COMMANDED his people to begin offering animal sacrifices as part of their highly organized corporate worship. The law, over time, became closely identified with this complex sacrificial system required under the Old Covenant. The writer of Hebrews referenced this system when arguing that, *"without the shedding of blood,"* forgiveness of sins is impossible (9:22). Animals *had* to be sacrificed (see Lev 16); God's atonement of sin depended on it.

---

1. https://www.poets.org/poetsorg/poem/road-not-taken.
2. See, for starters, Lev chapters 1 and 3.

Animal sacrifice was always more about the owner's heart[3] than the flavor of the meat roasting over the fire. God never accepted second best: sick, lame, inferior animals were totally repugnant to him (see Mal 1:8). Only strong, healthy animals *"without blemish"* (Lev 1:3) could be offered; only they represented a true sacrifice (pain and loss) to their owners. God essentially challenged the Israelites to bring their blue-ribbon winners, their most expensive animals (and offer them in the right way), or they would die in their sins.

Animals were slaughtered in staggering numbers under the Old Covenant. Fortunately, God no longer demands animal sacrifices. Now, worship that pleases his heart requires *human* sacrifice: the sacrifice of *all* of his people! New Covenant human sacrifices are, however, radically distinct from the animal sacrificial system. Under the Old Covenant, the sacrificed animals *died*. Now, by the tender *"mercies of God,"* believers are called to joyously sacrifice themselves and *live!* Paul phrased this new standard of worship, the one specifying *human* sacrifice, in these terms: *"I appeal to you therefore, brothers, by the mercies of God, to present your bodies as a living sacrifice, holy and acceptable to God, which is your spiritual worship"* (Rom 12:1).

Human sacrifice offered to God with gratitude: this defines the acceptable standard of worship under the New Covenant. We offer *"spiritual worship"* as we joyfully sacrifice our lives to him. Daily, our wills, pride, arrogance, self-serving motives must be "slaughtered" in sacrifice to the One who promised we can *"have life and have it abundantly"* (John 10:10). Paul's *"spiritual worship"* is not restricted to Dove-award-winning music, nor is it confined to cathedrals, centuries-old liturgies, or 75-minute mega-church worship services. Rather, spiritual worship most clearly occurs in those places requiring spiritual decisions about Christ's Lordship: the TV lounge, the kitchen, the gym, the office, even the supermarket. How many Christians would alter (rather, *altar!*) their shopping lists if Jesus accompanied them down the grocery aisles?

---

3. See "Worship that God Rejects (Malachi 1:6–14)."

True *"spiritual worship"* can occur in both the grocery store and the house of worship!

HUMAN SACRIFICE IN CHRISTIAN PERSPECTIVE

Paul certainly had a way with words! He may have honed this skill during all those hours studying while smelling Gamaliel's feet (Acts 22:3), or in response to the life-transforming anointing of the Holy Spirit (Acts 13:9–12). In any case, Philippians 3:18–19 illustrates brilliantly Paul's use of powerful word images: *"For many . . . walk as enemies of the cross of Christ. Their end is destruction, their god is their belly, and they glory in their shame, with minds set on earthly things."* Whoever these "enemies" were, they broke Paul's heart! Note that he did not describe them as "enemies of Christ"—rather, *"enemies of the cross."* The cross, for Paul, demanded *total* surrender to Christ's Lordship—in every arena of life, including food! With perfect comfort-crushing clarity, the cross speaks of death: to ungodly physical desires, to selfish ambition, to undisciplined appetites, and (in the context of Phil 3) to worshipping the "god" of the gut!

Eating contests[4] illustrate as poignantly as a 44-inch waist how bellies can become the focal point of human existence! Winners of such contests *"glory"* in their gluttonous shame. Abusing the bodies entrusted by their Maker, contestants worship their guts *"rather than the Creator, who is blessed forever"* (Rom 1:25). I am growing increasingly concerned about friends in the faith who would rather talk about their favorite restaurant than their Lord. How easily we can become seduced by our appetites! How easily we can begin worshipping our bellies and the food that fills them. How easily we can welcome a soft-and-comfortable, pain-free version of the gospel that opposes the central message of the cross of Christ Jesus!

TV's food and shopping channels cater endlessly to those whose minds (and appetites) are *"set on earthly things"* (Phil 3:19).

---

4. To say nothing of chug-a-lug beer-guzzling contests!

When Christians allow *any* physical appetite to dominate their lives, they invariably oppose the offensive message of the cross! Such believers creatively justify their wanton sensuality—especially so when their spiritual shepherds, often guilty themselves, never even mention such sins!

"MORE THAN THESE?" AN INVITATION TO SACRIFICIAL JOY

The lakeside chat recorded in John 21 must have been extraordinarily painful for Peter. First, his Lord privately asked Peter if he loved him (Jesus) *"more than these"* (see 21:15). What was Jesus referring to when posing this piercing question? The context suggests Jesus was motioning toward *"breakfast"* (21:12)—rather, its leftovers—or perhaps the 153 large fish being cleaned by eager fishermen on the shore. Jesus demanded that Peter love him more than breakfast, more than fish, more than fishing, more than any person, object, or practice that threatened to dull the impact of the cross!

Paul wrote one section of Philippians *"with tears"* (3:18) because those described in verse 19 had likely been, at one point, fellow believers. They had, apparently, been seduced by their earthly appetites—similar to the spiritual plants that spring up *"with joy"* on life's rocky soil in the parable of the sower and the seed (Matt 13:5–6, 20–21). Christ's reference to joy in that context differs greatly from the "painful joys" in this book's subtitle. *Rocky-soil* joy simply cannot last; its roots have not painfully pushed past (or through) the surrounding rocks. Such joy *will* wither! Only deeply rooted *sacrificial* joy can survive long-term.

THE JOYFUL ROAD "LESS TRAVELED BY"

A painful alternative route is available to the broad, well-travelled road on which many—both in and out of the Church—are travelling (Matt 7:13). Cardio training, strength training, and fasting partially pave that narrow, less-travelled road. Friendship with *"the cross of Christ"* (Phil 3:18) demands the sacrificial surrender of our comfort and will. It also demands the eager embrace of a disciplined life in which food serves the body, and the body serves the Holy Spirit as his temple. We *dare not* assume that a gluttonous, weak, and unfit body is *"holy and acceptable"* (Rom 12:1) to the Suffering Servant (Isa 53), who willingly bore the iniquity of us all.[5]

This small book has sought to challenge its readers to discover at a gut level (literally) what Paul meant about presenting our bodies as living sacrifices. Is my body *"holy and acceptable"* to God? Is yours? Imagine that I am suffering from one or more of the common *lifestyle-inflicted* diseases. Can I assume that I am getting this "living-sacrifice" business right? I think not. Living sacrifices have one Lord, and seek only to please him. They are drawn, like steel to a magnet, to his altar—daily.

"And that has made all the difference." Robert Frost's concluding line hints of some profound consequence of choosing "the road less traveled by." For those willing to walk the more demanding, often painful road of physical and spiritual discipline, their "human sacrifice" of time, effort, comfort, and food (when fasting) constitutes acceptable *"spiritual worship."* Such people know the joy created by self-sacrifice and full embrace of the cross of Christ. If you have not already joined them, may your future choices guide you to this road less travelled. Those choices can, indeed, make "all the difference."

5. This bold statement applies only to those who are physically-medically able to pursue physical fitness. *All* believers, however, even those with physical impairments, are called to pursue a disciplined life with regard to food intake and fasting.

APPENDICES

Appendix A

My Strength-Training Routine

CURRENT MEDICAL CONCERNS-CONDITIONS THAT IMPACT MY STRENGTH TRAINING

Upper spine and neck stiffness	I avoid dead lifts and any lift putting a load on top of my shoulders (e.g., standing toe-risers).
Right knee	I avoid conventional (bar across shoulders) deep squats and heavy-weight leg extensions.
Left shoulder (operated on in 2003)	I don't do overhead lat pull-downs, vertical press lifts, butterfly lifts, and chin-ups.

Note: See chapter 14: Pain 101.

STRENGTH-TRAINING WORKOUT: MONDAY AND FRIDAY

Lift	Sets: Reps	Current Weight	Notes
Pushups (Mondays: See Notes)	2 sets: 50*	Body weight only	Attempt 50 on the 2nd set
Crunches	1 set: 60+	Body weight only	On an exercise ball
Squats	2 sets: 50*	25 lb. plate weights	Against a wall using an exercise ball for support; one plate in each hand
Seated horizontal row	2 sets: 8 to 10	180 lbs.	160 lbs. on 2nd set
Calf extensions	2 sets: 20+	460 lbs.	[seated toe risers]
Seated curls	2 sets: 6 to 8	100 lbs.	80 lbs. on 2nd set
Horizontal leg curls	2 sets: 12	140 lbs.	120 lbs. on 2nd set
Seated chest press	2 sets: 8 to 10	170 lbs.	
Shoulder shrugs	2 sets: 12+	45 lb. plate weights	One in each hand
Crunches with oblique twist	1 set: 60+	Body weight only	On an exercise ball; left side then right
Incline back extension	1 set: 30+	Body weight only	
Shoulder rotations	2 sets: 12+	25 lbs.	Each arm; two angles 20 lbs. on 2nd set
Suspended knee lifts	1 set: 25+	Body weight only	
Lunges	2 sets: 14+	25 lb. plate weights	One in each hand

Notes: * I limit the first set to 50 reps, treating it as a warm up; I then max out the second set, trying for at least 50 reps: pushups, squats.

The symbol "+" means or more—depending on the day.

WEIGHTLESS WEDNESDAYS

Lift	Sets: Reps	Resistance Details	Notes
Planking: horizontal	1 set	Body weight only	1 min. 45 sec.
Left/right oblique dips	1 set: 25+	Body weight only	Side planking position
Planking: leg lifts	1 set: 20+ (each)	Body weight only	First left, then right
Crunches	1 set: 60+	Body weight only	On an exercise ball
Squats	2 sets: 50+	Body weight only (using an acute angle)	Against a wall using an exercise ball for support
Crunches with oblique twist	1 set: 60+	Body weight only	On an exercise ball
Incline back extension	1 set: 30+	Body weight only	
Shoulder rotations	2 sets: 12+	Thera-band resistance	Each arm; 2 distinct horizontal pull motions
Suspended knee lifts	1 set: 25+	Body weight only	
Lunges	2 sets: 14+	Body weight only	Focus on form, full extension of quad muscles

Note: The symbol "+" means or more—depending on the day.

Appendix B

Lord of All—Even My Fork

The Gospels and the Pauline epistles emphatically teach that the resurrected Christ is Lord of all. This foundational truth resounds throughout the New Testament, from his claim to *"all authority in heaven and on earth"* in Matthew 28:18 to the *"King of kings and Lord of lords"* emblazoned on him in Revelation 19:16. Because of this, we often admonish, "If Christ is not Lord of all, He is not Lord *at* all!"

Accepting his lordship requires that we accept his "unreasonable" demands (by the world's standards) on our lives: *"If anyone would come after me, let him deny himself and take up his cross daily and follow me"* (Luke 9:23). Living disciplined, moral lifestyles, we boldly declare that Christ is Lord. And we invite others to accept him as Lord, investing time and effort in those struggling to fully accept this paramount doctrine of the Christian life. Alcoholics, drug addicts, those trapped in pornography: such people burden our hearts as we counsel and pray for spiritual and physical break-throughs in their lives. We long for them to walk in the paradoxical freedom gained through submission to Christ. And then we go to lunch!

Ah, lunch! Delicious, captivating food. Once seated at the table of culinary delight, thoughts of Christ's lordship, self-denial, and taking up our cross daily quickly vanish. After all, we have first given thanks, asking God to bless the food to our bodies. So the more we eat, the more he can bless. And bless! And bless!

Do self-denial and cross-bearing apply to breakfast, lunch, and dinner? Until late November 2011, I had never even considered this question. Yet I was desperately discontent with my weight, overall health, and spiritual lethargy. Diets did not work, nor did self-initiated acts of my will: I frequently tried both. I often left restaurants feeling stuffed and totally defeated, picking up my small cross of daily self-denial at the front door where I had unthinkingly left it. This lordship-denying, restraint-free approach to dining is, sadly, the norm for many believers.

On December 1st, 2011, by God's intervening grace, I embraced a new style of living . . . and eating. Instead of consuming the "mandatory" three meals a day, I chose to let hunger determine the number of meals I ate. This normally meant eating half of a light breakfast at brunch and a modest evening meal. Nothing special was involved—no targeting of particular foods: everything in moderation. And only when truly hungry!

The spiritual insights I have gained regarding his comprehensive claims upon my life have been more impactful than the 90 pounds I have lost since December 2011. These insights have rocked my world, frequently leading to times of repentance for the decades of abuse I have inflicted on my body, the body he created to glorify him. The apostle Paul summarized powerfully his response to Christ's right to rule over every aspect of our lives: *"I will not be dominated by anything"* (1 Cor 6:12). To the extent that our appetites are out of control, food has mastered us! Just as our bodies are not meant for sexual immorality (1 Cor 6:13), they certainly are not meant for obesity and gluttonous indulgence.

Until late 2011, I effectively denied Christ's lordship over my appetite, struggling with obesity and private, personal defeat for most of my life as a result. My fork considered itself immune to Christ's radical claims. Now it, too, confesses—through its relative inactivity daily—that Jesus Christ is indeed Lord of all.

Appendix C

The Amazing ELF Diet

THE AMAZING ELF[1] DIET offers guaranteed weight loss, with no:

- pills
- injections
- purchase of special meals
- psychotherapy
- surgery
- gimmicks
- checklists
- calorie-counting hassles

ELF is highly effective . . . AND recommended by almost every doctor.

ELF will even save you money each month . . . LOTS of money in some cases!

Some people experience mild, uncomfortable side effects (hunger) during the first few weeks, but the benefits in health,

---

1. Eat Less Food

weight loss, and financial savings make the *copyright-free* ELF diet worth the effort and discomfort.

The ELF "Diet"

1. Eat only when hungry . . . *really* hungry. (This supersedes item 3 below.)

2. Eat nothing after 7:30 pm.

3. Eat two modest meals a day: brunch (from 10:30 am to 11:30 am) and dinner.

4. Eat only "firsts"—avoid going back for "seconds."

5. Brush your teeth right after dinner: this discourages late-night ELF cheating!

6. Limit carbs (e.g., bread): they make you feel *extra* hungry later.

7. Divide and conquer (cravings and stupid calories) when eating out. Request a carry-out box when you place your order. When served, immediately cut all food items in half; put one half in the box. After eating the remaining half, ask yourself if you are still hungry . . . *really* hungry. If not, you have tomorrow's evening meal ready to take home with you.

   Come to terms with eating take-away leftovers. (And spend less time cooking!)

   For the romantic-at-heart: go half-zies by sharing dessert, or even the entire meal. (And no take-away box is needed.)

8. Embrace mild hunger: it is not your enemy, but *can* be your weight-loss friend.

Food remaining on my plate after I am no longer hungry becomes a sacrifice to the Lord. May it be pleasing to him.

"I will not be dominated by anything." 1 Corinthians 6:12

Bibliography

"100 Million Dieters, $20 Billion: The Weight-Loss Industry by the Numbers." ABC News. Accessed August 26, 2018. http://abcnews.go.com/Health/100-million-dieters-20-billion-weight-loss-industry/story?id=16297197.

"4 Essential Spiritual Benefits of Physical Exercise." Jon Beaty. November 16, 2016. Accessed August 26, 2018. http://www.jonbeaty.com/4-essential-spiritual-benefits-of-physical-exercise/.

"5 Health Benefits of Doing Plank Exercise." Mercola.com. Accessed August 26, 2018. http://fitness.mercola.com/sites/fitness/archive/2014/12/05/5-plank-benefits.aspx.

"Aerobic vs. Anaerobic: What's Best for Weight Loss?" Healthline. Accessed August 26, 2018. http://www.healthline.com/health/fitness-exercise/aerobic-vs-anaerobic.

"BMI (Body Mass Index): What Is BMI?" Medical News Today. January 05, 2016. Accessed August 26, 2018. https://www.medicalnewstoday.com/info/obesity/what-is-bmi.php.

Brand, Paul, and Philip Yancey. *Pain: The Gift Nobody Wants*. London: Marshall Pickering, 1994.

"Cardio Exercise Definition and Benefits." HealthStatus. September 30, 2017. Accessed August 26, 2018. https://www.healthstatus.com/health_blog/wellness/cardio-exercise-definition-and-benefits/.

"Cardiovascular Exercise & Weight Loss." Super Skinny Me. November 11, 2012. Accessed August 26, 2018. http://www.superskinnyme.com/cardiovascular-exercise.html.

Cline, Krista M. C., and Kenneth F. Ferraro. "Does Religion Increase the Prevalence and Incidence of Obesity in Adulthood?" *Journal for the Scientific Study of Religion* 45, no. 2 (2006): 269–81. doi:10.1111/j.1468-5906.2006.00305.x.

Corleone, Jill. "How Much Weight Will I Lose on a Water Fast?" LIVESTRONG.COM. July 18, 2017. Accessed August 26, 2018. https://www.livestrong.com/article/221792-how-much-weight-will-i-lose-on-a-water-fast/.

Danielsson, Matt. "How to Calculate Your Heart Rate!" Bodybuilding.com. December 09, 2014. Accessed August 26, 2018. https://www.bodybuilding. com/fun/matt62.htm.

"Defining Adult Overweight and Obesity." Centers for Disease Control and Prevention. June 16, 2016. Accessed August 26, 2018. https://www.cdc. gov/obesity/adult/defining.html.

"Does Building Muscle Burn Fat, Calories & Increase Metabolism?" A Workout Routine. November 28, 2017. Accessed August 26, 2018. https://www. aworkoutroutine.com/does-building-muscle-burn-fat/.

Elkaim, Yuri. "This Resistance Band Workout Routine Will Get You Toned." Yuri Elkaim. June 29, 2018. Accessed August 26, 2018. https://yurielkaim. com/resistance-band-workout-routine/.

"Fasting and Fast-Days." JewishEncyclopedia.com. Accessed August 26, 2018. http://www.jewishencyclopedia.com/articles/6033-fasting-and-fast-days.

"Fat in Church." Fox News. Accessed August 26, 2018. http://www.foxnews. com/opinion/2012/06/03/obesity-epidemic-in-america-churches.html.

"Food Addiction." WebMD. Accessed August 26, 2018. https://www.webmd. com/mental-health/eating-disorders/binge-eating-disorder/mental-health-food-addiction#1.

"Food Opiates: Are You Addicted?" OAWHealth. June 05, 2018. Accessed August 26, 2018. https://oawhealth.com/2015/06/16/food-opiates-are-you-addicted/.

"Free Weights vs. Machines: Which Is Better?" BuiltLean. Accessed August 26, 2018. https://www.builtlean.com/2013/06/11/free-weights-vs-machines/.

"From Head to Toe: The Benefits of a Cardio Workout." Health Essentials from Cleveland Clinic. December 09, 2017. Accessed August 26, 2018. https:// health.clevelandclinic.org/2016/02/head-toe-benefits-cardio-workout-infographic/.

Garber, Carol Ewing et al. "Quantity and Quality of Exercise for Developing and Maintaining Cardiorespiratory, Musculoskeletal, and Neuromotor Fitness in Apparently Healthy Adults: Guidance for Prescribing Exercise." *Medicine & Science in Sports & Exercise* 43 (2011) 1334–59. doi: 10.1249/ MSS.0b013e318213fefb.

Genius, Stephen J. "Elimination of Persistent Toxicants from the Human Body." *Human and Experimental Toxicology* 30 (January 2011) 3–18. doi: 10.1177/0960327110368417.

"Gnosticism." Christianity.com. Accessed August 26, 2018. https:// www.christianity.com/church/church-history/timeline/1-300/ gnosticism-11629621.html.

"Great Lent." OCA. Accessed August 31, 2018. https://oca.org/orthodoxy/the-orthodox-faith/worship/the-church-year/great-lent.

Hansen, Mark Victor, and Robert G. Allen. *The One Minute Millionaire: The Enlightened Way to Wealth.* New York: Three Rivers, 2009.

Healy, Melissa. "Nearly 4 in 10 US Adults Are now Obese, CDC Says." The Columbus Dispatch. October 14, 2017. Accessed August 26, 2018. http://

www.dispatch.com/news/20171014/nearly-4-in-10-us-adults-are-now-obese-cdc-says.

Hewitt, Nathan. "10 Benefits of Fasting that Will Surprise You." Lifehack. August 06, 2018. Accessed August 26, 2018. http://www.lifehack.org/articles/lifestyle/10-benefits-of-fasting-that-will-surprise-you.html.

"How to Calculate Target Heart Rate Zone?" Polar USA. Accessed August 26, 2018. https://support.polar.com/us-en/support/How_to_calculate_target_heart_rate_zone_.

"Intermittent Fasting (Time-Restricted Eating)." Burnfatnotsugar.com. Accessed August 26, 2018. http://burnfatnotsugar.com/assets/if.pdf.

Kenny, Paul J. "Is Obesity an Addiction?" Scientific American. September 01, 2013. Accessed August 26, 2018. https://www.scientificamerican.com/article/is-obesity-an-addiction/.

Khazan, Olga. "The Second Assault." The Atlantic. December 15, 2015. Accessed August 26, 2018. https://www.theatlantic.com/health/archive/2015/12/sexual-abuse-victims-obesity/420186/.

Klein, A. V., and H. Kiat. "Detox Diets for Toxin Elimination and Weight Management: A Critical Review of the Evidence." *Journal of Human Nutrition and Dietetics* 28, no. 6 (2014): 675–86. Accessed August 26, 2018. doi:10.1111/jhn.12286.

"Latissimus Dorsi." The Free Dictionary. Accessed August 26, 2018. https://medical-dictionary.thefreedictionary.com/latissimus+dorsi.

Mack, Stan. "Is It a Myth that Muscle Burns More Calories than Fat?" LIVESTRONG.COM. July 18, 2017. Accessed August 26, 2018. http://www.livestrong.com/article/447243-is-it-a-myth-that-muscle-burns-more-calories-than-fat/.

Magee, Elaine. "8 Ways to Burn Calories and Fight Fat." WebMD. Accessed August 26, 2018. http://www.webmd.com/diet/obesity/features/8-ways-to-burn-calories-and-fight-fat#2.

"The Many Benefits of Fasting." AllAboutFasting. Accessed August 26, 2018. https://www.allaboutfasting.com/benefits-of-fasting.html.

"Maximum Heart Rate Formula." Dr. Gabe Mirkin on Health, Fitness and Nutrition. Accessed August 26, 2018. http://www.drmirkin.com/fitness/9156.html.

McCoy, William. "Can You Lose Weight with a 40-Minute Treadmill Workout?" LIVESTRONG.COM. September 11, 2017. Accessed August 26, 2018. https://www.livestrong.com/article/514587-can-you-lose-weght-working-out-40-minutes-on-the-treadmill/.

Miller, Paul. "7 Benefits of Doing Cardio for 30 Minutes a Day." Home Gym Heaven. November 22, 2017. Accessed August 26, 2018. http://homegymheaven.com/7-benefits-cardio-30-minutes-day/.

Nayak, Payal. "Behaviorism as a Theory of Personality: A Critical Look." Psychoanalysis: Freud's Revolutionary Approach. Accessed August 26, 2018. http://www.personalityresearch.org/papers/naik.html.

"Overweight & Obesity Statistics." National Institute of Diabetes and Digestive and Kidney Diseases, U.S. Department of Health and Human Services, August 01, 2017. Accessed November 08, 2018. www.niddk.nih.gov/health-information/health-statistics/overweight-obesity.

Persynaki, Angeliki et al. "Unraveling the Metabolic Health Benefits of Fasting Related to Religious Beliefs: A Narrative Review." *Nutrition* 35 (2017) 14–20. doi: 10.1016/j.nut.2016.10.005.

Ricketts, Donna. "What Is Aerobic Exercise? Definition, Benefits & Examples." Study.com. Accessed August 26, 2018. http://study.com/academy/lesson/what-is-aerobic-exercise-definition-benefits-examples.html.

Robergs, Robert A., and Roberto Landwehr. "The Surprising History of the HRmax=220-age Equation." *Journal of Exercise Physiology* 5 (May 2002) 1–10. Accessed August 26, 2018. https://eprints.qut.edu.au/96880/.

Salzberg, Steven. "Can a 3-day Fast Reset Your Immune System?" Forbes. December 30, 2014. Accessed August 26, 2018. https://www.forbes.com/sites/stevensalzberg/2014/12/30/can-a-3-day-fast-reset-your-immune-system/#15b5d0963c93.

Sarnataro, Barbara Russi. "Sore Muscles? Don't Stop Exercising." WebMD. Accessed August 26, 2018. http://www.webmd.com/fitness-exercise/features/sore-muscles-dont-stop-exercising#1.

Seliger, Susan. "Is Fasting Healthy?" WebMD. Accessed August 26, 2018. http://www.webmd.com/diet/features/is_fasting_healthy#2.

"Standing Calf Raises." Bodybuilding.com. Accessed August 26, 2018. https://www.bodybuilding.com/exercises/standing-calf-raises.

"Types of Fasting." AllAboutPrayer.org. Accessed August 26, 2018. http://www.allaboutprayer.org/types-of-fasting-faq.htm.

"Walk Your Way to New Blood Vessels." BIDMC Academy. Accessed August 26, 2018. https://www.bidmc.org/centers-and-departments/cardiovascular-institute/about-us/heartmail/heartmail-hot-topics/walk-your-way-to-new-blood-vessels.

Weil, Richard. "Aerobic and Anaerobic Exercise: Examples and Benefits." MedicineNet. Accessed August 26, 2018. https://www.medicinenet.com/aerobic_exercise/article.htm.

"What the $60 Billion Weight Loss Industry Doesn't Want You to Know." Washington Monthly. May 26, 2016. Accessed August 26, 2018. http://washingtonmonthly.com/2016/05/02/what-the-60-billion-weight-loss-industry-doesnt-want-you-to-know/.

"What's in Your Diet Pills?" @berkeleywellness. Accessed August 26, 2018. http://www.berkeleywellness.com/supplements/other-supplements/slideshow/what-your-diet-pills.

"Worship that God Rejects (Malachi 1:6–14)." Bible.org. Accessed August 26, 2018. https://bible.org/seriespage/2-worship-god-rejects-malachi-16-14.